BALANCE EXERCISES FOR SENIORS

Discover a Newfound Sense of Freedom with 100 Practical Exercises Tailored for Enhancing Senior Mobility and Stability

Payton Poling

Chapter 1: The Science of Balance

In the marvelous journey of life, balance truly is the unsung hero of our physical symphony, an intricate dance of muscles and mind that allows us to navigate the world with grace and stability. As we age, the importance of balance only grows, becoming a key player in our pursuit of an active and independent lifestyle.

Balance, at its essence, is the body's ability to maintain center of gravity over its base of support. This sounds simple enough, but it's a complex process involving several systems in our body working in harmony. Here, we'll explore what balance is, how it works, and its critical role in our daily lives.

The Inner Workings of Balance

Imagine balance as an experienced conductor managing a full symphony orchestra, where each musician represents a different system in our body. The conductor's baton guides three main 'instrumental sections': the sensory input systems, the brain, and the musculoskeletal system.

The Sensory Input - Roll Call of the Senses

Our bodies gather information about our position and movement through sensory organs, primarily our eyes, ears, and the proprioceptive system that senses the position of our limbs and joints.

Visual System: Our eyes act as the scouts, sending visual cues to the brain about our position concerning our environment. This is why closing your eyes while standing on one foot can be challenging. We rely heavily on what we see to keep us upright and navigate safely.

Vestibular System: Nestled deep within our ears, the vestibular system is the maestro of motion, it senses head movements and the pull of gravity. It keeps us upright during movement, telling us if we're tilting, turning, or standing straight.

Proprioception: This silent whisperer informs the brain about the body's position in space through nerve receptors in our muscles, tendons, and joints. Every time you take a step, proprioceptors in your feet and legs are hard at work, telling your brain where you are and what the ground beneath you feels like.

The Brain - Master of Ceremonies

The brain is the processing powerhouse where complex computations occur. It integrates all the input it receives from the sensory organs and, based on that, sends commands.

Integration: The brain operates like a high-speed computer, rapidly integrating sensory information to make sense of your position and movement.

Decision: Once the data is analyzed, the brain makes split-second decisions, instantaneously dispatching orders to various parts of the body to correct or maintain balance.

Learning and Memory: Think of this as the brain's library, filled with tomes of balance "instructions" from past experiences. The brain recalls and adapts these learned movements and responses to help keep you steady.

The Musculoskeletal System - Executors of Grace

Upon receiving the brain's directives, our muscles and joints act to either stabilize us or correct our balance.

Muscle Response: Muscles are our doers, responding rapidly to the brain's signals to contract or relax as needed to adjust the body's position.

Joint Coordination: Joints play a pivotal role, with their fluid movements allowing us to bend, twist, and turn without toppling over.

Strength and Flexibility: Robust muscles and flexible joints are fundamental for good balance. They provide the power and range of movement necessary to perform balancing acts.

Balance, Aging, and Adaptation

As we age, our concert of balance might face a few challenges. Parts of our sensory systems may not be as sharp as they once were; our muscles might lose some of their strength, and our joints may not be as supple. But here's the good news—our balance system can adapt. Like fine-tuning an instrument, we can improve our balance with practice.

Practical Insights from the Theory of Balance

Understanding how balance works lays the groundwork for appreciating the balance-enhancing exercises we'll explore later in this book. Here are some practical insights drawn from our theoretical understanding:

Stay Visually Vigilant: Keep your home well-lit and remove tripping hazards. Enhancing your visual environment aids your balance.

Ear Health Matters: Take care of your ear health, as issues here can directly impact your balance. If you experience dizziness or vertigo, consult with a healthcare professional.

Nourish Your Proprioception: Walking barefoot on various surfaces can boost the sensitivity of your proprioceptors. Safe, tactile exercises enhance this critical sense.

Challenge and Change: Just as musicians practice to perfect a piece, challenging your balance in controlled ways can help fine-tune it. Repeating movements and balance exercises can train your system to respond more effectively.

Muscle Power: Strength-building exercises are not merely for aesthetics; they are vital for maintaining balance. Lower body strength, in particular, equates to better stability.

Flex for Success: Flexibility declines with age, but it doesn't have to be that way. Regular stretching and mobility exercises can ensure your joints stay limber, supporting better balance.

Mind Your Medications: Some medications can affect your balance. Be informed about your prescriptions, and if necessary, discuss alternative options with your healthcare provider.

In Conclusion: A Lifelong Pursuit

The quest for better balance is not a one-time event; it's a lifelong pursuit. And it's worth every effort. The grace and stability that come with a well-tuned balance system open up a world of activities and independence. It allows you to enjoy the golden years with confidence and poise, whether you're strolling through a park, dancing at a grandchild's wedding, or simply moving through your daily routines.

Connecting the theory to practical application, we can now begin to understand the grand performance of balance and how it supports our everyday actions. As Payton Poling, I invite you to join me in exploring simple yet effective exercises designed to improve your balance. Empower yourself through understanding and action. After all, every step you take with assured balance is a step towards an active, independent life filled with opportunity and joy.

1.2 Age-Related Changes in Balance and Stability

As we age, our bodies undergo a multitude of changes—our vision may soften around the edges, our hearing might not be as sharp, and our memory can play tricks on us. One area of change that often goes overlooked, yet is fundamentally significant to our daily lives, is our sense of balance. Balance is an intricate system involving a harmonious interaction between the brain, muscles, bones, and sensory systems, and like the finest of symphonies, it requires each component to perform impeccably. The road of time, however, can introduce a few obstacles along the way.

The changes in balance and stability we experience as we age are as natural as the wrinkles upon our skin, yet they carry their own unique challenges. It's crucial to understand what happens inside our bodies—the unseen dance of physiology and time.

As we gracefully step into our senior years, various physiological changes can make maintaining balance a tad more challenging. The interplay between how we perceive the world around us and how we move within it, shifts. On a foundational level, there are several systems within our body that contribute to our dynamic sense of balance and stability: the vestibular system (including inner ear function), vision, proprioception, muscle strength, and reaction time.

The vestibular system, our internal gyroscope, begins to decline in function, a bit like the winding down of a beautifully crafted watch. This can lead to a sense of dizziness or vertigo, a sensation which none of us are fond of. Our vision, which acts as a guide to our environment, may become less sharp. As a result, it might become harder to navigate through a world that now seems slightly out of focus. This challenge is compounded at night or in poorly lit areas, as our eyes take longer to adapt to changes in light.

Proprioception, our body's natural knowledge of where it is in space, relies on signals sent from sensory nerves in our muscles and joints. This internal map of our bodies can become less detailed, leaving us a little more uncertain of our footing. Muscle mass and strength often decrease too, leading us onto a path where we might not feel as steady on our feet as we once did. The strength we draw upon to stand upright, to walk with confidence, and even to sit down gracefully becomes diminished.

Furthermore, our reaction time slows down. The speed with which we adjust our movements to avoid tripping over an unexpected obstacle isn't quite as swift. Each of these factors alone can influence our balance, but often they conspire together, creating a perfect storm that can make our steps more tentative.

Often misunderstood is the intertwining relationship between balance and the broader musculoskeletal system. Our bones, the frame upon which our bodies rest, lose density over time, a condition known as osteoporosis. This makes them more fragile and susceptible to fractures, adding a potential risk when balance is lost. Joint health, too, comes into play. Conditions such as arthritis cause discomfort and can restrict our range of motion, both of which contribute to our overall ability to maintain and correct balance when off-kilter.

The golden years should be a time of celebration, reflection, and enjoyment. So, it is only fitting that we acknowledge how these changes can impact not just our physical selves but our mental and emotional well-being. When we notice a change in our balance, a common response is fear—a fear of falling, which can become quite profound. This fear may close us off from engaging in activities we love or from attempting new experiences.

Our bodies, those steadfast companions through the years, can begin to feel unfamiliar which can be unsettling, even frustrating. A chance stumble or a missed step can suddenly shake our confidence. However, like a seasoned navigator, we find solace and surety in understanding these changes. This knowledge becomes our compass, pointing us toward the appropriate precautions and adaptations we can make.

Adapting does not mean surrendering to age; it means embracing it with intelligence and poise. Consider the small acts we can integrate into our daily routine, for instance, wearing proper footwear that offers support and reduces the risk of slips; ensuring our living spaces are well-lit—like setting the stage for our continued performance; and removing trip hazards from paths we frequently tread. Simple measures—all woven into the fabric of our day-to-day lives—can significantly bolster our balance and stability.

The crux of the matter is this: while age-related changes in balance are an inevitable part of life's journey, they are not insurmountable hurdles. They're simply new rhythms to learn and incorporate into the dance we call living.

Through the chapters to come, we will embark on a journey together, full of practical exercises and movements designed specifically for the senior body—one that may be experiencing these natural shifts in balance and stability. We will explore ways to reawaken and strengthen those systems within us that contribute to a centered, stable existence. Where we find limitation, we will seek adaptation, ensuring that each step, turn, and reach is performed not only with safety in mind but with a spirit of renewed freedom as well.

The coming pages are your guide. Together we will discover the key elements of balance, tailor our approach to meet your unique needs, and, most importantly, we will walk hand in hand toward a future where each step is taken with confidence and grace.

In closing, let us remember, like a tree that sways in the wind yet remains deeply rooted, we too can learn to bend gracefully with the ebb and flow of time, maintaining our balance and standing tall amidst the changing seasons of life. Welcome to the journey.

The intricacies of balance often go unnoticed until they begin to falter. This invisible thread that weaves through our daily movements becomes startlingly apparent when its reliability is questioned. For seniors, this realization often comes hand in hand with a cascade of psychological effects that can weigh heavily on daily life.

Understanding the psychological impact of balance issues requires empathy and a deeper appreciation for how these concerns interlace with our sense of self and security. The narrative of movement is not just physical—it's a story that evolves with our emotions, confidence, and cognitive health.

The Understated Narrative of Balance

Balance is like an unsung hero—the quiet backdrop to every step we take. It's only when its steadiness is threatened that we notice the crucial role it plays. For seniors, the decline in balance can be a source of worry that whispers caution with every movement. The fear of falling, one of the most common concerns among the senior population, can transform open spaces into obstacle courses and familiar routines into challenges fraught with potential danger.

Research has illuminated this darker side of balance issues: an increased risk of depression, anxiety, and social withdrawal. As balance wanes, so too can our luminescence, dimming the enthusiasm we once had for activities we cherished. The silent struggle against a wavering balance can cast a shadow on life's simple pleasures—walking in the park, dancing at a family wedding, or even navigating the kitchen to brew a pot of morning coffee.

The Ripple Effect of Decreased Confidence

Confidence and balance have a symbiotic relationship. When balance falters, confidence often tumbles alongside it. This relationship holds significant sway over a senior's autonomy. The activities that once spoke to a person's independence can become sources of trepidation. No longer buoyed by the certainty of secure footing, seniors may retreat into shells of inactivity, magnifying their feelings of vulnerability.

In this context, the psychological impact can manifest as a reluctance to engage in social gatherings, a hesitancy to participate in physical activities, and an overarching sense of frailty that undermines self-assuredness. From a psychological standpoint, it is as if the ground beneath one's feet has not just become unsteady—it has turned into something akin to quicksand, slowly eroding self-reliance and quality of life.

Cognitive Considerations and Balance

Cognitive function and balance maintain an intricate dance within our neurology. Our mind's health is a patchwork quilt of memories, skills, and abilities, all of which can be tenderly linked to balance. As we age, cognitive decline may accompany balance issues, and these intertwined changes can play their tune on mental wellbeing.

An apt illustration is seen in how spatial awareness and the planning of movement come together to allow us to navigate our world. When balance is impaired, the cognitive load increases, demanding more attention to avoid tumbling. This heightened state of alertness can be mentally exhausting, leaving less cognitive bandwidth for other pursuits. Over time, this mental fatigue can contribute to a decline in cognitive vitality, making it increasingly challenging to stay engaged and mentally sharp.

The Social Spin of Balance

The tapestry of human connection is rich with threads of shared experiences. Balance issues can unravel these connections as seniors begin to shy away from activities that foster camaraderie and communion. The simple joy of walking to a neighbor's house for tea might become a mountainous trek, filled with trepidation at the thought of a misstep.

This pullback from society feeds loneliness, and the encroaching isolation can lead to a profound sense of disconnection. Humans are social creatures, and the absence of interaction can lead to palpable declines in mental health—inflicting a loneliness that is as harmful to longevity as smoking or obesity.

Resilience and Adaptation

Despite these challenges, the human spirit is a resilient marvel, capable of adapting to change with grace and determination. Finding balance, both physically and psychologically, often involves embracing new strategies for movement and wellbeing. Adaptation might mean learning to trust again—trust in oneself, trust in others, and trust in the environment.

Part of adaptation is the empowerment that comes from recognizing and combating the psychological effects of balance issues. By confronting these challenges head-on, seniors can reweave the threads of their confidence and reinstate their place in the social tapestry that enriches their lives.

Harnessing a Positive Outlook

A positive outlook can be a powerful antidote to the adverse psychological effects of balance issues. It is about shifting the focus from what has been lost to what can be gained. Encouraging activities that foster a sense of achievement, providing opportunities for social engagement, and supporting avenues for laughter and joy can help rebuild the confidence that balance issues so often erode.

Practical Pathways Forward

The intersection of psychological support and balance training opens up a practical pathway for seniors facing these issues. An understanding that balance exercises not only improve physical steadiness but also fortify mental fortitude provides a dual-purpose approach. With professional guidance, seniors can engage in exercises that are not only beneficial for their physical health but also fundamentally supportive of their mental and emotional wellbeing.

In this journey, success is measured not by the elimination of fear, but by the courage to face it. Each small triumph in stability can reverberate through the psyche, lifting the spirits and nurturing the soul. It is this harmonious blend of physical and psychological support that can help seniors rediscover their footing, both in the literal and metaphorical sense.

In the realm of balance, there is much that remains unseen—forces that ebb and flow beneath the surface of our consciousness. Yet by shining a light on the psychological impact of balance issues, we can begin to understand the full spectrum of these challenges and, in turn, offer guidance, comfort, and, most importantly, a pathway forward that is grounded in empathy and emboldened by hope.

2.1 ASSESSING YOUR CURRENT BALANCE ABILITY

Embarking on a journey of balance training beams like the first ray of dawn—it ushers in new possibilities and the promise of steadier days. As we tenderly age, our physical landscape shifts, and like a seasoned navigator recalibrating their compass, it's essential to assess where we currently stand. Acquainting ourselves with our balance ability is akin to planting our feet firmly on the ground before a gentle leap forward.

Balance is far more than not tipping over; it's an intricate collaboration of muscles, senses, and reflexes. To appraise it effectively, begin with understanding that each person's starting point is a tapestry woven from years of unique experiences. As such, being honest with oneself is paramount. After all, the landscape of our bodies hides no secrets from us.

A self-assessment, when approached methodically, can be deeply enlightening. Let's unfold the parchment to draw the map of our present.

The Cornerstones of Balance Ability

Balance is underpinned by a few key systems: our vision, inner ear vestibular system, and proprioceptors—sensors within our muscles and tendons that tell us our position in space. Each cog in this machine needs to turn smoothly.

To evaluate our balance, a quiet, safe environment is essential. A sturdy chair or countertop nearby, to grasp hold of, should our trustworthy steadiness momentarily falter, is wise. Comfortable clothing that does not restrict movement allows for honest exploration of our capabilities.

Initial Self-Observation

Starting with an observation may seem elementary, yet there is no substitution for it. Observe how you walk; do you feel a sway or a hitch in your step? When you stand, do you wobble or feel the need to shift weight frequently? How often do you reach out for support from objects around you? These initial observations are fundamental precursors to a more structured assessment.

Structured Self-Assessment Techniques

Once you've attuned to the general quality of your balance, the next step is to put it to a gentle test. Here are a few structured techniques to consider:

Single-Leg Stance: Stand near your support object, lifting one foot an inch above the ground. How long can you hold the position without touching down or needing support? Try this on both legs.

Heel-to-Toe Walk: Similar to a tightrope walk but on solid ground, practice walking in a straight line, placing the heel of one foot directly in front of the toe of the other. Does it feel like an act in a circus, or do you move with the grace of a seasoned performer?

The Reach Test: From a standing position, extend your arm and lean forward or to the side, reaching as far as possible without losing your footing. Feel that edge where stability meets the void of imbalance.

Standing Up from a Chair: Do you need to thrust your body forward with momentum or is a graceful rise possible? The ability to stand smoothly speaks volumes about strength and balance.

Walking Assessment: Pace your usual walk. Is it slow and measured, or do you manage to carve out a rhythm that speaks of confidence and ease?

Each attempt at these assessments will not only evaluate your balance but will also subtly start training your ability. It's a dance of discovery and an embrace of hope.

Standardized Balance Assessments

Standardized tests, which clinicians and fitness professionals commonly use, can also be employed here, albeit with care and simplicity. While not exhaustive, a few examples include:

Timed Up and Go (TUG) Test: Measure the time it takes to stand up from a seated position, walk a set distance (usually around 10 feet), turn around, walk back, and sit down again. The shorter the time, the better the functional mobility.

30-Second Chair Stand Test: Determine how many times you can stand from a seated position and sit back down in 30 seconds. This offers insight into the coordination between balance and strength.

Reflect, Document, Repeat

Each time these tests are performed, insights reveal themselves. Write them down. Keep a balance journal. The very act of documenting adds a tangible presence to your progress, and it becomes a narrative of growth. Note not only the metrics but also how you felt. Were you tense, or did calm confidence keep your company?

When performing these assessments, it is vital not to overexert. Safety comes first, always. Moreover, the aim is not to tilt full force towards mastery in one go. Balance, like the finest single-malt whiskey, is better when it matures slowly.

Embracing Your Baseline

There's no place for judgment here. Wherever your initial assessment lands, it is a starting point, neither good nor bad. It's the mark from where you can stride ahead. If the attempts seemed like whispers of a bygone era when balance was taken for granted, worry not. Even whispers can be nurtured into songs.

Consulting with Professionals

After self-assessment, you might consider consulting with healthcare providers or fitness professionals, especially if concerns about your equilibrium arise. They can perform more sophisticated assessments and guide you towards exercises entirely tailored to your current abilities.

Crafting Your Path

Understanding where your balance stands today is the groundwork upon which you can construct a castle of stability. The exercises, practical advice, and steps forward in this book are designed to be adaptable—they will meet you at your current ability and gallantly travel with you on this journey.

In Conclusion

No matter how tranquil or tempestuous the seas of assessment are, remember, these are waters that can be navigated with patience and persistence. Recognize your balance ability, respect your starting point, and relish the voyage ahead. From here, every step, every shift, every rise, is a step toward a future of confidence and independence where the fear of falling recedes like the tide and a newfound sense of freedom arises.

Embarking on a journey to improve balance and stability can be as liberating as it is necessary, especially for seniors who long to maintain their autonomy and joy in everyday activities. As we prepare our bodies and minds for balance training, it is essential to plant our feet firmly in the soil of realistic expectations. This grounding will not only nourish our efforts but also help us flourish as we progress.

When setting out to enhance your balance through exercise, it is critical to acknowledge where you're starting from. Assessing your current balance ability, as we discussed previously, gives us a baseline. From there, we must set goals that are attainable, considering your unique circumstances. Goals that are too lofty may become overwhelming and disheartening, while goals set too low may not provide enough challenge to stir improvement.

Think of goal setting as plotting a course on a map; you need to know your destination, understand the terrain, and plan for stops along the way. It's about balancing ambition with ability, and progression with patience.

First and foremost, identify the 'why' behind your goals. Are you aiming to walk more safely to the mailbox? Perhaps you'd like to feel more confident standing and chatting with friends, or you might long for the gratification of completing household tasks independently. Whatever your 'why', let it be the compass that guides your objectives.

In setting these goals, consider SMART criteria, a method often hailed for its effectiveness in various aspects of life—from business management to personal development. Each goal should be Specific, Measurable, Achievable, Relevant, and Time-bound.

A **Specific** goal is direct and pinpointed: "I want to improve my balance so I can stand on one foot for at least 10 seconds."

A **Measurable** goal allows you to track progress: "I'll practice my standing exercises three times a week and record my times."

An **Achievable** goal takes into account your personal capabilities and limitations: "Given my current stability, aiming to achieve this in two months is realistic."

Make sure it's **Relevant** to your personal aspirations and lifestyle: "Improving my balance will help me engage more confidently in community yoga classes, which is a passion of mine."

And lastly, being **Time-bound** provides a sense of urgency and a deadline: "I will reach this goal in eight weeks."

Moreover, be kind enough to yourself to understand that it's okay to adjust these goals as you go along. Progress in balance, as in life, is not always linear. It may ebb and flow, and your aspirations might need to shift to accommodate that rhythm. Pacing yourself is not a concession; it's intelligent strategy.

Now, let's explore some foundational milestones that can act as rungs on the ladder toward your overarching goals.

First Milestone: Mastering Static Exercises. Before you conquer the dynamics of motion, stand still. Can you sit without support? Stand with your feet together? These are essential first steps, and achieving them will build a sense of accomplishment.

Second Milestone: Introducing Movement. After mastering stillness, add simple movements. Lifting an arm, turning your head, or lifting a heel are movements that condition your body to maintain balance during activity.

Third Milestone: Progressing to Dynamic Balance. This is where you begin to walk, step sideways, and perhaps step backward under controlled conditions. It's about learning to find your center as your body moves through space.

Fourth Milestone: Incorporating Dual Tasks. Dual-tasking involves performing a cognitive task while balancing, such as counting backward from 100 while standing on one foot. This simulates real-life scenarios where you must think and move simultaneously.

As you progress through these milestones, revel in each achievement. Balance training is not only physical; it's psychological. Your confidence will grow with each small victory, and this buoyancy will push you through moments of stagnation or setback.

Take heart in the fact that improvements in balance and stability can be felt even when they're not immediately visible. Maybe you'll notice less wobbling while brushing your teeth or an improved steadiness when navigating a crowded room. Don't overlook these subtle signs; they're harbingers of the progress that's unfolding.

Prepare your environment to facilitate your training. Create a safe space where you can practice without fear of falling. Consider investing in sturdy handrails, non-slip mats, and adequate lighting. An environment tailored to safety will not only protect you but also empower you.

Embrace the idea of incremental improvement. Rome wasn't built in a day, and balance can't be perfected in a single session. Sometimes, a one-second improvement in standing on one foot is as monumental as it is motivational. Resist the temptation to compare yourself to others. Your journey is your own, and your goals should reflect that singularity.

Finally, let's touch on the emotional elements of setting goals. It's natural to feel daunted or discouraged at times. When these feelings arise, lean on your support network—family, friends, caregivers, or community members. Share your goals and celebrate each step forward with these allies.

Remember, setting realistic goals and expectations isn't about limiting your potential; it's about harnessing it. By planting your feet on the solid ground of viable objectives, establishing a clear and achievable path, and arming yourself with patience and support, you will discover a newfound sense of freedom. As you strengthen your muscles and mind for the journey of balance training, carry with you the knowledge that each step taken is a stride toward greater independence and vitality.

Creating an environment conducive to safe balance practice is akin to preparing for a voyage. The intent is not merely to embark on a journey, but to do so with assurance and safety as unwavering companions. As you set sail into the rewarding waters of balance exercises, let's cultivate a habitat that not only minimizes risk but also fosters a sense of security that paves the way for progress and wellbeing.

A Foundation of Stability

Safety begins underfoot. Exercise on a flat, non-slip surface—be it carpet, a yoga mat, or a specialized no-slip flooring solution. Ensure the texture of the surface is gentle yet grippy, safeguarding against slips that could lead to falls.

Adequate Space

Freedom to move entails ample space. As we mature, our steps may become more cautious, but our movements should not be constrained by clutter. Clear your practice area of any furniture or objects that could pose a tripping hazard. Ample room allows for free motion and eliminates the mental distraction over potential obstacles.

Good Lighting

Clarity of vision ensures clarity of action. Excellent lighting allows you to be aware of your surroundings and move confidently. Reduce shadows and glares that might distort perception and contribute to an unstable gait.

Appropriate Footwear

A solid foundation starts with what encases the foot. Slippery socks can spell disaster as much as ill-fitting shoes. Choose footwear that snugly hugs the foot, providing ample arch support and a non-slip sole, or opt for barefoot when safe to do so, which can improve the sensory connection to the floor.

Supportive Equipment

Stability aids stand ready at your beck and call. Have a sturdy chair or countertop nearby to grip if balance wanes. Other tools such as handrails or walking aids should be at hand, particularly for exercises that challenge your balance more significantly.

Investing in Assistive Tools

Advanced tools are not symbols of weakness, but instruments of strength. Simple assistive devices such as a rubber anti-fatigue mat can provide additional support and comfort, particularly during standing exercises.

Distraction-Free Zone

Concentration is the bedrock of practicing balance. Minimize distractions in your environment. Television, radio, and other noise can divert attention from the body's signals. Foster a zone of tranquility where focus meets intention.

Uninterrupted Time

Allocate a time when interruptions are least likely. Consistency not only builds a habit but ensures that the time you set aside for practice is protected. Cell phones can wait; this is a time for self-care, not for device care.

Attire for Success

Comfort in clothing translates to confidence in movement. Wear loose, comfortable clothing that does not restrict your range of motion or alter your sense of balance. This immersion encourages a connection to the exercises and heightens your awareness of body positioning.

Personalize Your Space

A personal touch adds comfort and familiarity. Integrate elements that have meaningful connections, such as photos, soft music, or plants. These create a nurturing environment, turning your practice space into a personal sanctuary for wellbeing.

Creating the Correct Mental Space

Setting the stage physically is just as important as preparing the mind. Before delving into each session, take a few deep breaths, and allow yourself to become present in the moment. A positive mindset lays the groundwork for a responsive body.

Accessibility

Consider the journey to and from the practice area. The path should be free of tripping hazards and should accommodate any supportive devices used. Room transitions, such as doorway thresholds, should be examined for potential risks. The safer the access, the more likely the consistency in practice.

Temperature Control

Comfort is not solely about the tactile or visual. The right temperature can make a significant difference in your motivation to practice. Too cold, and muscles may stiffen; too hot, and discomfort might discourage activity. Aim for a temperature that is warm enough to encourage muscle pliability without causing overheating.

Reflective Feedback

Mirrors can serve as a silent guide. If possible, use a full-length mirror during practice to observe alignment and posture. This real-time feedback promotes self-correction and heightens body awareness while offering visual affirmation of your hard work.

In Case of Emergency

Hope for the best, plan for the worst. Have a phone accessible in case of an emergency, and consider wearing a medical alert system if living alone or possessing certain health conditions. Informing a family member or friend about your exercise routine imbues an added layer of safety.

Consistency in Location

The consistency of space reinforces the habit. Designate a specific area for your balance practice to cultivate an association with exercise. This repetition evokes a pavlovian response, where the mere sight of this space triggers a readiness to engage in your routine.

Your Audience

If company is preferred, invite it. A trusted relative, friend, or caregiver can provide encouragement, and if necessary, physical support. A session observed is often a session improved, as it fosters accountability and camaraderie.

Embrace Modifications

Listen to the body's dialogue with the chosen environment. If something feels off, be open to altering the set-up. Adaptations are not regressions; they are prudent adjustments that align practice with current capacities.

Psychological Safekeeping

Recognize that the setting is not solely a protector of the body but a guardian of the psyche. A space drenched in safety is like a warm embrace from an old friend—it allows the mind to engage fully, without the whisper of worry about potential harm.

Gradual Challenges

Progress follows patience. As confidence breeds within your safe zone, slowly introduce minor changes to your environment that present calculated challenges to your balance—intentional, not impulsive, all the while keeping safety paramount.

The environment you forge is a reflection of the respect you hold for your body in its pursuit of balance. Small touches of forethought—non-skid rugs, reachable supports, a clear path—imbue every action with intention and imbibe each movement with meaning. May your practice space be a testament to your commitment to safety, a canvas where the art of balance is both honed and celebrated with each step taken and each breath exhaled.

Chapter 3: Basic Balance Exercises

As we embark on the journey to enhance balance and stability, seated exercises offer a safe starting point for seniors seeking to maintain their mobility and prevent falls. This collection of exercises is designed with the physical capabilities and safety considerations of older adults in mind. Each routine is meticulously crafted to challenge and improve balance from the comfort and security of a chair, providing a low-risk environment to build strength and confidence. The exercises will range from gentle isometrics to dynamic movements that engage various muscle groups—all pivotal for a strong and stable foundation. Let's begin the path toward a balanced and independent life with these empowering seated stability exercises.

Seated Marching

Objective of the Exercise: To improve lower body strength and coordination from a stable seated position.

Difficulty Level: Beginner

Equipment Needed: A sturdy chair without wheels.

Description:

- Sit upright in the chair with feet flat on the floor.
- Slowly lift one knee toward the chest as high as comfortable, then place it back down.
- Alternate legs as if marching in place, ensuring a controlled movement with each lift.

Key Focus Points:

- Maintain an erect posture throughout the exercise.
- Focus on lifting the knee using the muscles in your thigh and hip.
- Engage your core muscles to aid balance.

Benefits:

- Strengthens the hip flexors and quadriceps.
- Enhances coordination which is critical for walking and climbing stairs.
- Stimulates concentration and cognitive function through rhythmic movement.

Variations and Adaptations:

- Add ankle weights for increased resistance.
- Perform the exercise with one hand lifted to enhance core engagement.

Frequency and Duration: Perform for 1-2 minutes, once or twice daily.

Seated Side Taps

Objective of the Exercise: To engage the oblique muscles and promote lateral stability.

DIFFICULTY LEVEL: Beginner

EQUIPMENT NEEDED: A sturdy chair without wheels.

DESCRIPTION:

- Sit in the chair with your back straight and feet flat.
- Tap one foot to the side as far as comfortably possible, then bring it back to center.
- Alternate sides, maintaining an upright torso and engaging the obliques as you tap.

KEY FOCUS POINTS:

- Keep shoulders relaxed and back straight.
- Use the abdominals to stabilize your body.
- Breathe out as you tap to the side and in as you return to center.

BENEFITS:

- Develops lateral core strength.
- Improves balance during side-to-side movements.
- Aids in stabilizing the pelvis.

VARIATIONS AND ADAPTATIONS:

- Increase the range of movement as flexibility improves.
- Tap the foot to a slightly elevated object for added difficulty.

FREQUENCY AND DURATION: Perform 10 taps per side, twice daily.

UPPER BODY TORSO TWISTS

OBJECTIVE OF THE EXERCISE: To strengthen the core muscles and increase torso mobility.

DIFFICULTY LEVEL: Beginner

EQUIPMENT NEEDED: None.

DESCRIPTION:

- Sit upright with feet planted on the floor.
- Place hands on your shoulders or extend your arms out to the sides.
- Gently twist your torso to the right as far as comfortable, then to the left, keeping hips and legs facing forward.

KEY FOCUS POINTS:

- Engage core muscles during the twist.
- Move slowly and control the motion to prevent over-twisting.
- Keep your chin aligned with your chest to avoid neck strain.

BENEFITS:

- Improves rotational flexibility of the spine.
- Strengthens abdominal and back muscles integral for posture.

- Reduces the risk of back pain.

VARIATIONS AND ADAPTATIONS:

- For added challenge, hold a lightweight object while twisting.
- Incorporate a gentle forward bend to engage different muscle groups.

FREQUENCY AND DURATION: Perform 10 twists to each side, once or twice daily.

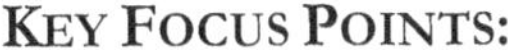

OBJECTIVE OF THE EXERCISE: To strengthen the arms and shoulders while increasing upper body stability.

DIFFICULTY LEVEL: Beginner

EQUIPMENT NEEDED: A sturdy chair without wheels.

DESCRIPTION:

- Sit on the edge of the chair with your feet planted firmly on the floor.
- Place your hands beside you on the seat of the chair.
- Push down into the chair to lift your body a few inches off the seat, then lower yourself back down.

KEY FOCUS POINTS:

- Keep your back close to the chair.
- Avoid straining your shoulders; move within a comfortable range.
- Engage your core to aid stability.

BENEFITS:

- Enhances arm and shoulder strength.
- Improves ability to lift oneself, assisting in getting in and out of chairs and beds.
- Builds upper body stability.

VARIATIONS AND ADAPTATIONS:

- To increase difficulty, extend one leg straight ahead.
- If full lift-off is too challenging, simply press down to engage the muscles without lifting.

FREQUENCY AND DURATION: Perform 8-10 push-ups, once or twice daily.

OBJECTIVE OF THE EXERCISE: To strengthen the muscles in the lower legs and feet, crucial for balance.

DIFFICULTY LEVEL: Beginner

EQUIPMENT NEEDED: None.

DESCRIPTION:

- Sit with a straight back and feet flat on the floor.

- Shift your weight to your heels and lift your toes up as high as you can.

- Then, shift to your toes and lift your heels.

KEY FOCUS POINTS:

- Keep your upper body still and use your legs to perform the movement.

- Focus on smooth transitions from heel to toe.

- Keep your hands on your thighs or the arms of the chair for stability.

BENEFITS:

- Improves strength and flexibility in the feet and ankles.

- Encourages circulation in the lower extremities.

- Aids in walking and navigating uneven surfaces.

VARIATIONS AND ADAPTATIONS:

- Try lifting only one foot at a time for a singular focus.

- Introduce a soft resistance band for added strength training.

FREQUENCY AND DURATION: Perform this rocking motion for 1-2 minutes, once or twice daily.

SEATED KNEE EXTENSIONS

OBJECTIVE OF THE EXERCISE: To improve strength in the quadriceps, which are essential for leg stability.

DIFFICULTY LEVEL: Beginner

EQUIPMENT NEEDED: None.

DESCRIPTION:

- Sit upright with feet flat and hands resting on the thighs.

- Extend one leg out in front until it is parallel to the ground, if possible, then lower it back down.

KEY FOCUS POINTS:

- Ensure back is not arching during the exercise.

- Squeeze the quadriceps at the top of the movement.

- Move in a slow and controlled manner to prevent jerking.

BENEFITS:

- Builds quadriceps strength for better support in standing and walking.

- Engages the core for improved stability while seated.

VARIATIONS AND ADAPTATIONS:

- Add ankle weights for extra resistance.

- If full extension is too challenging, extend the leg only partially.

FREQUENCY AND DURATION: Perform 12-15 extensions for each leg, once or twice daily.

OBJECTIVE OF THE EXERCISE: To enhance flexibility in the torso and improve range of motion for daily tasks.

DIFFICULTY LEVEL: Beginner

EQUIPMENT NEEDED: A sturdy chair without wheels.

DESCRIPTION:

- Sit upright with feet planted.
- Raise one arm overhead.
- Lean gently to the opposite side, using your other arm to hold onto the chair for support.

KEY FOCUS POINTS:

- Ensure you're stretching through the side of your torso and not twisting.
- Keep your movements fluid and avoid any jerky motions.
- Return to an upright position before switching sides.

BENEFITS:

- Promotes better flexibility in the sides of the body.
- Helps with reaching and bending activities.
- Assists in maintaining a straighter posture.

VARIATIONS AND ADAPTATIONS:

- Increase the stretch by leaning slightly further as flexibility improves.
- Use a small, soft ball to squeeze overhead for added upper body engagement.

FREQUENCY AND DURATION: Hold each stretch for 15-20 seconds, repeat 2-3 times per side, once daily.

In this section of "Simple Standing Balance Routines," we dive into the foundational practices that help forge a path toward enhanced balance and stability. Each routine is carefully crafted to respect the limitations and harness the capabilities of seniors, aiming to steadily build confidence and physical steadiness. The significance of these exercises lays not just in preventing falls, but in nurturing the everyday freedom that balance affords, allowing for a more active and joyful daily life.

WEIGHT SHIFTS

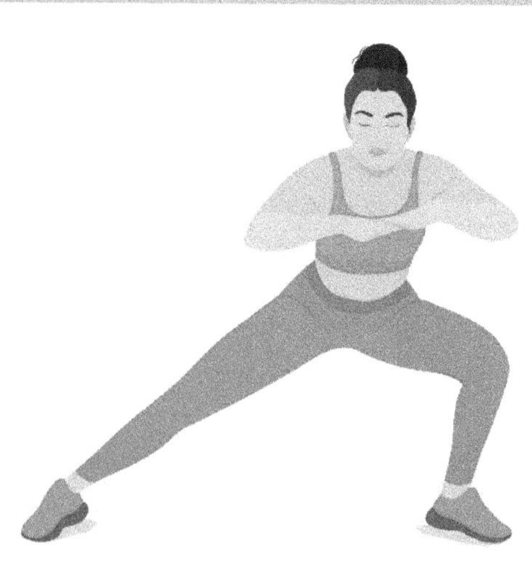

OBJECTIVE OF THE EXERCISE: To gradually improve balance by shifting weight from one leg to the other.

DIFFICULTY LEVEL: Beginner

EQUIPMENT NEEDED: No equipment needed.

DESCRIPTION:

- Stand with your feet hip-width apart and arms at your sides.
- Shift your weight onto your right leg, lifting your left foot just a few inches off the floor.
- Hold the position for up to 30 seconds, then gently place your left foot back on the floor.
- Repeat on the other side.

KEY FOCUS POINTS:

- Key Focus Points: Keep your supporting knee slightly bent.
- Engage your core muscles to help maintain balance.
- Breathe evenly throughout the exercise.

BENEFITS:

- Benefits: Promotes unipedal stance tolerance.
- Heightens proprioceptive awareness.
- Strengthens the supportive leg muscles.

VARIATIONS AND ADAPTATIONS:

- Variations and Adaptations: Hold onto a chair for added support.
- To increase difficulty, close your eyes while balancing.

FREQUENCY AND DURATION: Frequency and Duration: Perform 3 sets of 10-15 seconds holds per leg, 3-4 times a week.

OBJECTIVE OF THE EXERCISE: To increase hip flexor strength and coordination, enhancing the ability to walk and perform daily tasks safely.

DIFFICULTY LEVEL: Beginner

EQUIPMENT NEEDED: No equipment needed.

DESCRIPTION:

- Stand tall with your feet hip-width apart.
- Slowly lift your right knee towards your chest, as high as comfortably possible, keeping your back straight.
- Lower your leg and repeat with the left knee.
- Continue the "march" by alternating knees.

KEY FOCUS POINTS:

- Key Focus Points: Focus on lifting your knees using your hip muscles, not just momentum.
- Maintain an upright posture throughout the exercise.
- Keep your movements controlled and steady.

BENEFITS:

- Benefits: Develops coordination and hip flexor strength.
- Encourages safe walking mechanics.
- Activates core muscles for improved stability.

VARIATIONS AND ADAPTATIONS:

- Variations and Adaptations: Hold on to a countertop or the back of a chair for more stability.
- Increase the pace to challenge coordination.

FREQUENCY AND DURATION: Frequency and Duration: Perform for 1-2 minutes, two times a day.

OBJECTIVE OF THE EXERCISE: To strengthen the leg muscles and core while incorporating upper body movement for added stability challenge.

DIFFICULTY LEVEL: Intermediate

EQUIPMENT NEEDED: No equipment needed.

DESCRIPTION:

- Begin by standing on one leg, ensuring your non-supporting foot is clear of the ground.
- Slowly raise both arms to shoulder height in front of you.
- Maintain the position as long as you can comfortably manage, then lower your arms and switch legs.

KEY FOCUS POINTS:

- Key Focus Points: Keep a slight bend in the standing knee to avoid locking it.

- Maintain a straight posture with shoulders relaxed.

- Focus on smooth arm movements.

BENEFITS:

- Benefits: Encourages full-body coordination and balance.

- Strengthens the ankle and foot of the supporting leg.

- Develops core stability and upper body control.

VARIATIONS AND ADAPTATIONS:

- Variations and Adaptations: Perform the arm raise to the side or overhead to vary the challenge.

- Begin with shorter durations and progress as your stability improves.

FREQUENCY AND DURATION: Frequency and Duration: Hold for up to 30 seconds per leg, with 2-3 repetitions, every other day.

SIDEWAYS WALKING

OBJECTIVE OF THE EXERCISE: To enhance lateral movement agility and improve stability when shifting weight side-to-side.

DIFFICULTY LEVEL: Beginner

EQUIPMENT NEEDED: No equipment needed.

DESCRIPTION:

- Stand with your feet together and step to the side with your right foot.

- Bring your left foot to meet your right, maintaining a continuous motion.

- Take several steps in one direction, then return moving to the left.

KEY FOCUS POINTS:

- Key Focus Points: Keep your head up and look straight ahead.

- Engage your abdominal muscles for core support.

- Step smoothly and at a controlled pace.

BENEFITS:

- Benefits: Increases lateral hip strength and stability.

- Improves balance during sideways movements, helpful in navigating crowds and tight spaces.

VARIATIONS AND ADAPTATIONS:

- Variations and Adaptations: For more support, do this exercise next to a wall or while lightly holding onto a countertop.

- To increase difficulty, step over a small obstacle.

FREQUENCY AND DURATION: Frequency and Duration: Walk sideways for 10-15 steps in each direction, performing 2-3 sets, every other day.

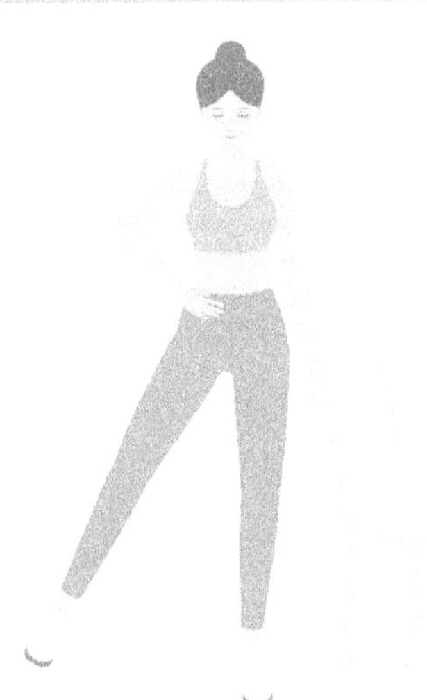

OBJECTIVE OF THE EXERCISE: To strengthen the muscles on the outer thigh and hips, which are crucial for lateral movement and balance

DIFFICULTY LEVEL: Beginner

EQUIPMENT NEEDED: None

DESCRIPTION:

- Stand behind a chair, placing hands lightly on the backrest for support.
- Shift your weight to one foot, keeping that leg slightly bent.
- Slowly lift the other leg out to the side, keeping it straight, then lower back down with control.

KEY FOCUS POINTS:

- Ensure weight is distributed evenly through the standing foot.
- Avoid leaning too much into the chair; use it only for light support.
- Keep the lifted leg straight and movements smooth and controlled.

BENEFITS:

- Increases hip mobility and strength, which is key for maintaining balance during side-to-side movements.
- Can help correct muscle imbalances and prevent falls.

VARIATIONS AND ADAPTATIONS:

- For a challenge, try performing the exercise without holding onto a chair, only using it as needed for balance.
- To modify, decrease the height of the leg lift.

FREQUENCY AND DURATION: Perform 10-15 lifts per leg, repeat 2-3 times on each side, once a day.

OBJECTIVE OF THE EXERCISE: To simulate walking in a straight line, enhancing balance and coordination

DIFFICULTY LEVEL: Beginner

EQUIPMENT NEEDED: None

DESCRIPTION:

- Stand straight and place your right foot directly in front of your left foot so your heel touches your toe.
- Take a step forward with your left foot, placing your heel directly in front of the toe of your right foot.
- Continue this heel-to-toe motion as if you are walking on a tightrope.

KEY FOCUS POINTS:

- Focus on a point ahead to keep your head and neck aligned and to maintain balance.

- Engage your core throughout the movement.

- Move in a slow and deliberate manner, concentrating on the heel-to-toe contact.

BENEFITS:

- Promotes a sense of spatial awareness and coordination.

- Helps improve stride patterns and gait, contributing to fall prevention.

VARIATIONS AND ADAPTATIONS:

- For a greater challenge, perform the exercise by looking from side to side instead of directly ahead.

- Use a hallway or a line on the floor as a guide if necessary.

FREQUENCY AND DURATION: Practice this walk for 5-10 feet and repeat 2-3 times, once or twice daily.

SINGLE-LEG STAND

OBJECTIVE OF THE EXERCISE: To improve balance and strength in the supporting leg and ankle

DIFFICULTY LEVEL: Moderate

EQUIPMENT NEEDED: None

DESCRIPTION:

- Stand with feet hip-width apart and near something sturdy you can hold onto if needed.

- Lift one foot slightly off the ground, balancing on the other leg.

- Hold the position while keeping your body upright and hips level.

KEY FOCUS POINTS:

- Keep your focus on a point directly ahead for balance.

- Engage the core muscles to maintain stability.

- Breathe evenly and resist the urge to hold your breath.

BENEFITS:

- Strengthens the ankles, legs, and core muscles, all of which are critical for good balance.

- Enhances focus and stability, reducing the likelihood of falls.

VARIATIONS AND ADAPTATIONS:

- For added challenge, try closing your eyes or turning your head side to side while balancing.

- To modify, keep your toes of the lifted foot on the ground and gradually increase the time the foot is in the air.

FREQUENCY AND DURATION: Hold for 10-30 seconds on each leg, repeat 2-3 times per session, once or twice a day.

Transitional movements form a bridge between static balance exercises and more dynamic activities. These exercises focus on smooth shifts from one position to another, enhancing the body's ability to respond to changes in balance. The essence of transitional movements is to replicate day-to-day motions, such as getting out of bed or reaching for an item on a shelf, in a controlled and safe exercise environment. By practicing these exercises regularly, seniors can strengthen their muscles and improve their reaction times, fostering greater autonomy and safety in their daily lives.

HEEL-TO-TOE STAND

OBJECTIVE OF THE EXERCISE: To enhance coordination and stabilize gait through controlled foot placement.

DIFFICULTY LEVEL: Beginner

EQUIPMENT NEEDED: None

DESCRIPTION:

- Begin by standing upright.
- Place the heel of one foot just in front of the toes of the other foot, as if walking on a tightrope.
- Hold this heel-to-toe position for a count of 20-30 seconds.
- Slowly shift to place the other foot in front and hold again.

KEY FOCUS POINTS:

- Focus on maintaining a straight posture throughout the exercise.
- Gaze forward to assist with balance.
- Use a wall or sturdy furniture for support if needed.

BENEFITS:

- Promotes steadiness during walking.
- Encourages precision in foot placement, crucial for navigating narrow spaces.

VARIATIONS AND ADAPTATIONS:

- To make it more challenging, try performing the exercise with eyes closed.
- To simplify, stand with feet side-by-side rather than in line.

FREQUENCY AND DURATION: Practice this exercise 5 times with each foot, once a day.

SIDE-TO-SIDE WEIGHT SHIFT

OBJECTIVE OF THE EXERCISE: To build lateral stability and strengthen the muscles used for side stepping.

DIFFICULTY LEVEL: Beginner

EQUIPMENT NEEDED: None

DESCRIPTION:

- Starting with feet slightly wider than shoulder-width apart, shift your weight to one side, bending the knee slightly as the other leg straightens.
- Return to the center and then shift to the opposite side, creating a smooth rocking motion.

KEY FOCUS POINTS:

- Keep your upper body straight and look ahead.
- Engage your core to maintain control.
- Shift weight as far as comfortable without straining.

BENEFITS:

- Enhances hip flexibility and leg strength.
- Improves balance for side-to-side movements, important for activities like getting into a car.

VARIATIONS AND ADAPTATIONS:

- Add arm movements that mimic the natural sway of arms while walking for a full-body exercise.
- If balance is an issue, perform near a countertop to hold onto for support.

FREQUENCY AND DURATION: Perform this exercise for 1 minute, twice a day.

SIT-TO-STAND WITH TURNS

OBJECTIVE OF THE EXERCISE: To improve the coordination between sitting, standing, and turning motions.

DIFFICULTY LEVEL: Intermediate

EQUIPMENT NEEDED: A sturdy chair without wheels.

DESCRIPTION:

- Sit in the middle of the chair, feet flat and arms crossed over the chest.
- Stand up, rotate your upper body to one side, then sit back down with control.
- Repeat on the other side.

KEY FOCUS POINTS:

- Ensure the transition from sitting to standing is steady and controlled.
- Keep the abdomen engaged.
- Turn head and shoulders together to enhance balance.

BENEFITS:

- Strengthens leg muscles and core.
- Improves ability to turn safely, reducing the risk of falls when changing directions.

VARIATIONS AND ADAPTATIONS:

- To decrease difficulty, use your hands for support during the sit-to-stand motion.

- Increase difficulty by holding a light object like a pillow during the turn.

FREQUENCY AND DURATION: Complete 6-8 repetitions on each side, once or twice a day.

OBJECTIVE OF THE EXERCISE: To synchronize lower and upper body movements, enhancing overall balance.

DIFFICULTY LEVEL: Beginner

EQUIPMENT NEEDED: None

DESCRIPTION:

- Stand with feet shoulder-width apart.
- Step forward with one foot and raise both arms in front, parallel to the floor.
- Hold the position briefly, then step back and lower arms.
- Alternate feet with each step.

KEY FOCUS POINTS:

- Keep your back straight and arms at shoulder height.
- Ensure your stepping foot lands firmly before lifting arms.
- Breathe evenly throughout the exercise.

BENEFITS:

- Encourages stability when switching between different poses.
- Strengthens the coordination between arm and leg movements.

VARIATIONS AND ADAPTATIONS:

- Increase the holding time of each step for added difficulty.
- Use elastic bands or light hand weights to strengthen arms.

FREQUENCY AND DURATION: Perform 8-10 steps with each foot, once a day.

OBJECTIVE OF THE EXERCISE: To improve ability to reach backward safely and maintain balance during everyday tasks.

DIFFICULTY LEVEL: Beginner

EQUIPMENT NEEDED: None

DESCRIPTION:

- Stand with feet hip-width apart.
- Shift your weight onto your front foot.
- Slowly reach one arm backward at shoulder height while extending the opposite leg back just above the ground.

- Return to the starting position and repeat with the opposite limbs.

KEY FOCUS POINTS:

- Concentrate on a focal point ahead to keep balance.
- Ensure the supporting leg is slightly bent.
- Move slowly to maintain control throughout the exercise.

BENEFITS:

- Strengthens the posterior chain.
- Improves proprioception for safer reaching in multiple directions.

VARIATIONS AND ADAPTATIONS:

- To reduce difficulty, perform the exercise near a wall for support.
- Add light ankle weights to the extended leg for increased strength training.

FREQUENCY AND DURATION: Complete 5-8 repetitions with each arm-leg combination, twice a day.

SINGLE-LEG STAND WITH TOE TOUCH

OBJECTIVE OF THE EXERCISE: To develop the ability to balance on one leg while performing a controlled reaching movement.

DIFFICULTY LEVEL: Intermediate

EQUIPMENT NEEDED: None

DESCRIPTION:

- Start in a standing position, shift your weight onto one leg, and lift the other leg's knee to hip level.
- Hinge forward at the hip and reach toward the toes of the lifted leg with the opposite hand.
- Hold briefly, then return to the initial single-leg stand.

KEY FOCUS POINTS:

- Keep the standing knee soft to avoid locking it.
- Use the hand not reaching for balance if needed.
- Keep movement slow and controlled to maintain form.

BENEFITS:

- Improves single-leg balance.
- Aids in bending and reaching movements without loss of balance.

VARIATIONS AND ADAPTATIONS:

- To simplify, touch the shin or knee instead of toes.
- Gradually progress to reaching lower as flexibility improves.

FREQUENCY AND DURATION: Aim for 5 repetitions on each leg, once a day.

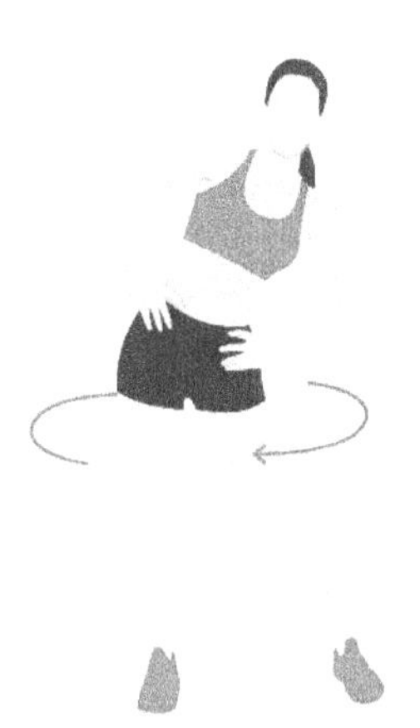

OBJECTIVE OF THE EXERCISE: To enhance hip mobility and build stability through circular hip movements.

DIFFICULTY LEVEL: Beginner

EQUIPMENT NEEDED: None

DESCRIPTION:

- Stand with feet shoulder-width apart and hands on hips.
- Lift one foot slightly off the ground and slowly move the leg in a circular motion, keeping the hip the pivot point.
- Alternate directions and then switch to the other leg.

KEY FOCUS POINTS:

- Keep the supporting leg steady and slightly bent.
- Maintain an upright posture.
- Move the leg in a controlled, smooth circle.

BENEFITS:

- Promotes hip flexibility.
- Strengthens muscles responsible for lifting the leg and stabilizing the core.

VARIATIONS AND ADAPTATIONS:

- Add a resistance band around the lower thighs to increase resistance.
- Perform while seated to reduce the balance challenge.

FREQUENCY AND DURATION: Complete 4-6 circles in each direction for both legs, once a day.

DOWNLOAD YOUR HOLIDAY BONUS

30 outdoor exercises of 3 levels of difficulty

If you found the recommended exercises helpful in improving your body performance, we would be very grateful if you could leave a review. Your feedback means a lot to us

CHAPTER 4: CORE STRENGTHENING FOR BETTER BALANCE

The core is the foundation of stability, and for seniors, a strong core facilitates balance and reduces the risk of falls. Core-focused seated exercises offer a secure platform for enhancing core strength without the risk of standing workouts. The exercises compiled here are crafted to engage various core muscles in a seated position, making them accessible to individuals with varying mobility levels. These routines are intended to enhance the overall stability and support necessary for daily functions, from turning to reach for an item to maintaining an upright posture.

SEATED MARCHES

OBJECTIVE OF THE EXERCISE: To activate the core muscles by lifting the legs alternately while seated.

DIFFICULTY LEVEL: Beginner

EQUIPMENT NEEDED: A sturdy chair without wheels.

DESCRIPTION:

- Sit upright in the middle of the chair with feet flat on the floor.
- Engage your core as you lift your right knee toward your chest, then lower it back to the starting position.
- Repeat the same movement with your left leg.
- Continue to alternate legs, ensuring to keep the core engaged throughout the movement.

KEY FOCUS POINTS:

- Focus on sitting up straight and engaging the core.
- Avoid using momentum; lift your legs with control.
- Breathe evenly and avoid holding your breath.

BENEFITS:

- Strengthens lower abdominals and hip flexors.
- Encourages better posture and balance.
- Increases circulation to the lower extremities.

VARIATIONS AND ADAPTATIONS:

- To increase difficulty, add ankle weights or pause and hold each leg in the lifted position for a count of three.
- For those with limited leg strength, perform smaller lifts.

FREQUENCY AND DURATION: Perform for 1-2 minutes, twice a day.

SEATED PELVIC TILTS

OBJECTIVE OF THE EXERCISE: To engage and strengthen the abdominal muscles by tilting the pelvis.

DIFFICULTY LEVEL: Beginner

EQUIPMENT NEEDED: None.

DESCRIPTION:

- Sit upright at the edge of the chair with feet firmly on the ground.

- Without moving your shoulders or feet, tilt your pelvis forward to flatten your lower back, then tilt backward to arch it slightly.

- Engage your core muscles to control the movement and keep your spine neutral.

KEY FOCUS POINTS:

- Keep movements smooth and controlled.

- Concentrate on isolating the pelvic movement without overarching the back.

- Maintain even breathing throughout.

BENEFITS:

- Improves lower back flexibility and strength.

- Enhances awareness and control of pelvic and abdominal muscles.

VARIATIONS AND ADAPTATIONS:

- For a challenge, pause and hold the tilt position for a few seconds.

- To adapt, those with lower back issues should reduce the range of motion.

FREQUENCY AND DURATION: Perform 10 tilts, twice a day.

SEATED SIDE BENDS

OBJECTIVE OF THE EXERCISE: To strengthen the oblique muscles on the sides of the abdomen.

DIFFICULTY LEVEL: Beginner

EQUIPMENT NEEDED: None.

DESCRIPTION:

- Sit upright with feet flat on the ground and arms hanging by your sides.

- Slowly bend to the right, sliding your right hand down towards the knee, then return to the center.

- Repeat the move on the left side.

- Alternate sides, engaging the core to maintain posture.

KEY FOCUS POINTS:

- Keep your buttocks in contact with the seat.

- Ensure you are bending directly to the side, not diagonally forward or back.

- Keep your head aligned with your spine.

BENEFITS:

- Targets obliques which improve lateral stability.

- Aids in the performance of daily activities involving side bending or twisting.

VARIATIONS AND ADAPTATIONS:

- Introduce a hand weight in one hand to increase resistance.
- For those who need to adapt, reduce the range of motion by bending less.

FREQUENCY AND DURATION: Perform 8-10 bends per side, twice a day.

SEATED OBLIQUE TWISTS

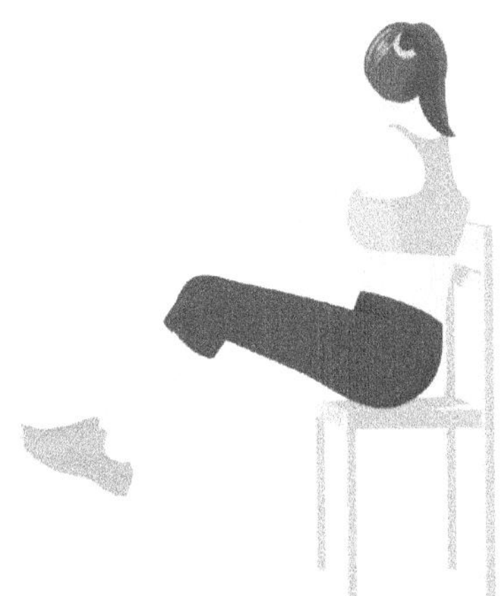

OBJECTIVE OF THE EXERCISE: To target the rotational strength and coordination of the core muscles.

DIFFICULTY LEVEL: Intermediate

EQUIPMENT NEEDED: A light medicine ball or a small pillow.

DESCRIPTION:

- Sit upright in the chair with feet flat and hold a medicine ball or pillow at chest level with both hands.
- Rotate your torso to the right, moving the ball to the side, then rotate to the left.

KEY FOCUS POINTS:

- Engage your core throughout the rotation.
- Keep your hips and legs facing forward.
- Coordinate your breathing with your movements - exhale on twist, inhale on return.

BENEFITS:

- Strengthens the oblique muscles.
- Encourages thoracic mobility.
- Improves rotational movements essential for daily tasks.

VARIATIONS AND ADAPTATIONS:

- For added difficulty, hold the twist for a few seconds before rotating to the opposite side.
- To adapt, use no weights and reduce the rotation range.

FREQUENCY AND DURATION: Perform 10 twists to each side, twice a day.

SEATED FORWARD PRESS

OBJECTIVE OF THE EXERCISE: To engage the abdominal wall and improve posture and frontal core stability.

DIFFICULTY LEVEL: Beginner

EQUIPMENT NEEDED: A light resistance band or a towel.

DESCRIPTION:

- Sit upright with feet grounded and hold the resistance band in front of you with both hands, elbows bent.
- Straighten your arms, pushing the band forward while squeezing your abdominal muscles.
- Return to the starting position with control.

KEY FOCUS POINTS:

- Keep your shoulders down and back.
- Resist the band's pull to maintain control.
- Breathe out as you press forward and in as you return.

BENEFITS:

- Strengthens the core stabilizers and shoulders.
- Improves postural support.
- Enhances functional movements like pushing doors.

VARIATIONS AND ADAPTATIONS:

- Increase the band's resistance for a greater challenge.
- If lacking mobility, perform the exercise without the band, extending just the arms.

FREQUENCY AND DURATION: Perform 12-15 presses, twice a day.

SEATED LEG EXTENSIONS

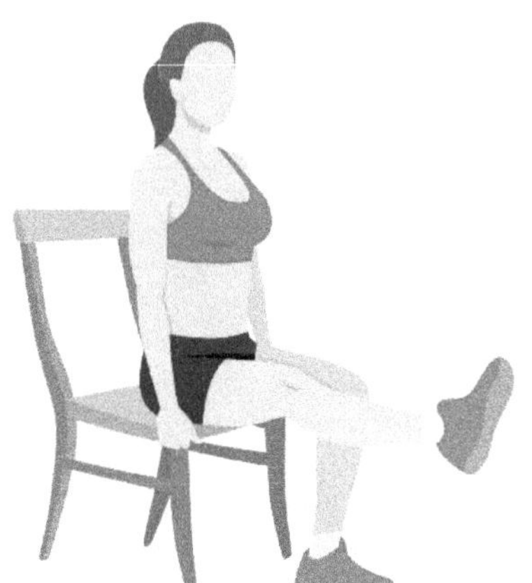

OBJECTIVE OF THE EXERCISE: To reinforce the quadriceps and core simultaneously while in a seated position.

DIFFICULTY LEVEL: Beginner

EQUIPMENT NEEDED: None.

DESCRIPTION:

- Sit with your back straight and feet flat on the floor.
- Extend one leg out in front of you as straight as possible, hold it there briefly, then lower it back to the floor and repeat with the other leg.

KEY FOCUS POINTS:

- Focus on maintaining a tall posture throughout the exercise.
- Squeeze the quadriceps at the top of the movement.
- Avoid locking your knee when extending your leg.

BENEFITS:

- Builds quadriceps and core strength.
- Promotes functional leg control and stability.
- Enhances coordination between upper and lower body.

- Add ankle weights for increased resistance.
- For those with knee issues, limit the extension range to keep a slight bend in the knee.

FREQUENCY AND DURATION: Perform 10-12 extensions per leg, twice a day.

SEATED ELBOW TO KNEE CRUNCHES

OBJECTIVE OF THE EXERCISE: To improve core endurance and coordination between the upper and lower body.

DIFFICULTY LEVEL: Intermediate

EQUIPMENT NEEDED: None.

DESCRIPTION:

- Sit on the edge of the chair and lean back slightly.
- Bring one knee up as you bring the opposite elbow down towards the knee, gently twisting the body.
- Return to the starting position and alternate sides.

KEY FOCUS POINTS:

- Ensure you twist your torso while keeping your buttocks on the chair.
- Avoid jerky movements; use your core muscles to control the motion.
- Coordinate your breath with the movement—exhale on the twist.

BENEFITS:

- Boosts abdominal and oblique strength.
- Enhances cross-body coordination.
- Simulates daily activities like reaching across the body.

VARIATIONS AND ADAPTATIONS:

- Increase the speed or add a pause at the top of the crunch for a challenge.
- For adaptation, perform the exercise without the elbow touching the knee, just moving them toward each other.

FREQUENCY AND DURATION: Perform 8-10 crunches per side, twice a day.

4.2 STANDING CORE STRENGTHENING ROUTINES

Welcome to a world where stability and vigor coexist in harmony, where each routine you embark upon empowers you with a robust core and the freedom to move assuredly. This specific segment of your journey is dedicated to standing core strengthening exercises, designed for enhancing your balance and stability from the ground up. These routines will focus on engaging various muscle groups within the core, which include your abdominals, pelvic muscles, back, and hips – the very epicenter of your physical well-being. With movements crafted to fit the contours of your life, these exercises are your stepping stones to an invigorated sense of self.

PELVIC TILT STAND

PELVIC TILT STAND

OBJECTIVE OF THE EXERCISE: To strengthen the lower back and abdominal muscles while improving posture.

DIFFICULTY LEVEL: Beginner

EQUIPMENT NEEDED: None.

DESCRIPTION:

- Start with your feet shoulder-width apart and your knees slightly bent
- Gently tuck your pelvis under, contracting the lower abdominal muscles, as if trying to flatten your lower back against an imaginary wall
- Hold this position for a few seconds, then slowly release and return to the starting position
- Keep your upper body relaxed and breathe evenly throughout the movement.

KEY FOCUS POINTS:

- Keep your movements slow and controlled
- Focus on engaging your core muscles during the tilt
- Maintain a relaxed breathing pattern.

BENEFITS:

- Improves core muscle stability which is critical for balance and back health
- Reinforces proper posture and alignment.

VARIATIONS AND ADAPTATIONS:

- To increase difficulty, perform the tilt with one foot slightly lifted off the ground
- For those with reduced mobility, perform the exercise near a counter or stable surface for support.

FREQUENCY AND DURATION: Repeat for 10-12 reps, 2-3 sets daily.

STANDING OBLIQUE CRUNCH

OBJECTIVE OF THE EXERCISE: To strengthen the oblique muscles for improved lateral stability and core strength.

DIFFICULTY LEVEL: Intermediate

EQUIPMENT NEEDED: None.

DESCRIPTION:

- Stand with your feet hip-width apart and your hands placed lightly behind your head
- Contract your core muscles and tilt to the right, aiming to bring your elbow towards your hip
- Return to the center, then repeat on the left side

- Focus on using your obliques to create the movement rather than your arms or legs.

KEY FOCUS POINTS:

- Ensure movements are controlled by the obliques
- Avoid pulling on your head or neck
- Keep hips stable and facing forward to isolate the core muscles.

BENEFITS:

- Targets side abdominal muscles, improving overall core stability
- Aids in the prevention of side-to-side falls by enhancing lateral balance.

VARIATIONS AND ADAPTATIONS:

- To modify, place hands on hips instead of behind the head
- Advanced individuals can hold small weights in each hand to increase resistance.

FREQUENCY AND DURATION: Perform 10-15 crunches on each side, for 2-3 sets daily.

STANDING BICYCLE CRUNCH

OBJECTIVE OF THE EXERCISE: To activate the full range of core muscles, especially the abdominals and obliques, while also enhancing balance and coordination.

DIFFICULTY LEVEL: Intermediate

EQUIPMENT NEEDED: None.

DESCRIPTION:

- Stand with your feet hip-width apart and your hands behind your head
- Bring your right elbow towards your left knee as you lift the knee and twist your torso
- Return to the start and then do the same with your left elbow to right knee
- Alternate sides in a smooth, controlled cycling motion.

KEY FOCUS POINTS:

- Focus on bringing elbow and knee together through the power of your abs
- Keep your spine naturally aligned
- Balance on one leg briefly to engage the core fully.

BENEFITS:

- Helps to develop a strong midsection for improved balance and posture
- Increases flexibility and coordination between the upper and lower body.

VARIATIONS AND ADAPTATIONS:

- For less intensity, perform without the twist and lift knees alternately
- Increase the challenge by holding each position for a second longer.

FREQUENCY AND DURATION: Do 10-12 cycles on each side, for 2-3 sets daily.

OBJECTIVE OF THE EXERCISE: To strengthen the hip stabilizers and obliques, and improve balance and flexibility in the hamstrings.

DIFFICULTY LEVEL: Intermediate

EQUIPMENT NEEDED: None.

DESCRIPTION:

- Stand with feet shoulder-width apart
- Lift your right leg forward and hold it in the air
- Stretch both arms out to the sides at shoulder height
- Slowly hinge at the hips, touching your left hand to your right foot, while keeping your right arm lifted towards the ceiling
- Return to the starting position and repeat on the other side.

KEY FOCUS POINTS:

- Keep your lifted leg straight, but not locked, as you hinge
- Engage your core throughout the exercise for better stability
- Look up towards your raised hand to maintain balance.

BENEFITS:

- Improves flexibility in the hamstrings and lower back
- Strengthens core and enhances balance and stability during movement.

VARIATIONS AND ADAPTATIONS:

- To lessen the difficulty, don't touch foot and just reach toward the toes
- Use a small weight in the upper hand for a more advanced workout.

FREQUENCY AND DURATION: Perform 8-10 windmills per leg, for 2-3 sets daily.

OBJECTIVE OF THE EXERCISE: To engage and strengthen the core muscles, specifically targeting the abs and obliques, while promoting coordination.

DIFFICULTY LEVEL: Intermediate

EQUIPMENT NEEDED: A flat wall.

DESCRIPTION:

- Stand facing away from a wall, about two feet from it.
- Lean forward and place your palms flat against the wall at shoulder height and shoulder-width apart.
- Bring one knee towards the wall as if you were attempting a mountain climber on the ground.
- Return that leg to the starting position and repeat with the other knee.
- Continue alternating legs in a smooth, controlled motion.

KEY FOCUS POINTS:

- Engage your core throughout the movement to maintain balance.
- Keep your movements measured and deliberate to avoid any jerking motions.
- Breathe steadily, exhaling as you bring each knee up.

BENEFITS:

- Strengthens core muscles aiding in balance and stability.
- Encourages coordination between upper and lower body movements.
- May help in improving posture.

VARIATIONS AND ADAPTATIONS:

- To reduce the difficulty, step back further from the wall, decreasing the body angle.
- For more intensity, incorporate a slight bounce on the supporting leg, akin to a light jog.

FREQUENCY AND DURATION: Aim for 2 sets of 12 reps for each leg, with a minute of rest in between, thrice a week.

CORE ENGAGED LEG LIFTS

OBJECTIVE OF THE EXERCISE: To strengthen the lower abdominal muscles and improve pelvic stability.

DIFFICULTY LEVEL: Beginner to Intermediate

EQUIPMENT NEEDED: None.

DESCRIPTION:

- Stand with your feet hip-width apart and your hands on your hips.
- Engage your core muscles and slowly lift one leg straight in front of you, without bending the knee.
- Hold this lifted position for a count of three.
- Slowly lower the leg back to the starting position and repeat with the other leg.

KEY FOCUS POINTS:

- Keep the standing knee slightly bent to avoid strain.
- Maintain an upright posture without leaning backward.
- Keep your core engaged throughout the lift to aid balance.

BENEFITS:

- Improves lower core strength, enhancing stability during walking and standing tasks.
- Reduces the risk of falls by improving control over leg movements.

VARIATIONS AND ADAPTATIONS:

- For those needing support, perform the exercise near a countertop or chair.
- Progress by holding the lifted leg for a longer duration or adding ankle weights.

FREQUENCY AND DURATION: Perform 10 lifts per leg, alternating, for two sets, four times a week.

OBJECTIVE OF THE EXERCISE: To fortify core stability by activating the abdominal and pelvic floor muscles.

DIFFICULTY LEVEL: Beginner

EQUIPMENT NEEDED: None.

DESCRIPTION:

- Stand erect with feet hip-width apart.
- Engage your core and pelvic floor muscles to tilt your pelvis slightly upward, flattening your lower back.
- Maintaining the pelvic tilt, lift one knee to hip level, then lower it gently.
- Alternate the lift with the opposite knee, as if marching slowly, while keeping your pelvis steady.

KEY FOCUS POINTS:

- Focus on engaging the pelvic floor muscles with each lift.
- Ensure your back stays flat throughout the exercise.
- Breathe evenly, coordinating your breath with your movements.

BENEFITS:

- Strengthens the lower abdomen and pelvic floor muscles.
- Promotes a stable and balanced gait.
- Encourages good posture and spinal alignment.

VARIATIONS AND ADAPTATIONS:

- To simplify, perform the exercise seated.
- Raise the intensity by holding the knee up for a longer count or adding a gentle twist towards the raised knee.

FREQUENCY AND DURATION: Complete 2 sets of 10 marches per leg, every other day.

4.3 DYNAMIC CORE STABILITY CHALLENGES

As we age, our core muscles are essential not just for good posture but also for maintaining balance and stability in our everyday movements. Dynamic core stability challenges are designed to engage not only the muscles of the abdomen and back but also those that support the entire trunk and pelvis area, contributing to an overall sense of steadiness and strength. In this section, we will explore a variety of exercises focused on enhancing core stability while also providing a moderate challenge for seniors who are ready to progress beyond basic core exercises.

OBJECTIVE OF THE EXERCISE: To engage and strengthen the core muscles through a dynamic passing motion

DIFFICULTY LEVEL: Intermediate

EQUIPMENT NEEDED: A lightweight medicine ball or a similarly sized ball

DESCRIPTION:

- Sit on a stability ball with your feet firmly planted on the floor and your spine straight
- Holding the medicine ball in both hands, slowly lean back without curving your spine, engaging your abdominal muscles
- Come back to the starting position and pass the ball to a partner or from one hand to the other, while maintaining your balance
- Repeat the pass while maintaining an upright and engaged core

KEY FOCUS POINTS:

- Focus on keeping your abdominal muscles tight throughout the exercise
- Keep your movements controlled and avoid any jerky motions
- Pass the ball at a moderate, manageable pace
- Ensure a steady breathing pattern

BENEFITS:

- Strengthens the abdominal and oblique muscles
- Promotes coordination and balance
- Encourages joint mobility in the arms and shoulders

VARIATIONS AND ADAPTATIONS:

- To modify, perform the exercise without a ball, simply mimicking the passing movement
- To increase difficulty, pass the ball in a figure-eight motion

FREQUENCY AND DURATION: Perform the pass for 1-2 minutes, once a day

STANDING OBLIQUE TWISTERS

OBJECTIVE OF THE EXERCISE: To target the oblique muscles and improve rotational stability

DIFFICULTY LEVEL: Intermediate

EQUIPMENT NEEDED: None

DESCRIPTION:

- Stand with your feet hip-width apart and your knees slightly bent
- Place your hands behind your head without pulling on your neck
- Rotate your upper body to the right, then to the left, initiating the movement from your waist
- Keep your hips stable and facing forward throughout the exercise

KEY FOCUS POINTS:

- Engage your core to protect your lower back

- Rotate only as far as comfortable without straining

- Focus on smooth, controlled movements

BENEFITS:

- Helps strengthen the oblique muscles crucial for twisting movements

- Encourages core stability and balance

- Enhances spinal flexibility

VARIATIONS AND ADAPTATIONS:

- For an easier version, perform the exercise seated on a chair

- To increase difficulty, hold a light weight in your hands while rotating

FREQUENCY AND DURATION: Perform 10-12 rotations on each side, 2 sets, every other day

PILATES SWIMMING

OBJECTIVE OF THE EXERCISE: To enhance coordination between the core and limb movements while engaging back muscles

DIFFICULTY LEVEL: Intermediate

EQUIPMENT NEEDED: Exercise mat

DESCRIPTION:

- Lie prone on an exercise mat with your arms extended in front of you and legs straight out

- Lift your right arm and left leg slightly off the ground, then alternate with your left arm and right leg, as if swimming

- Keep your head and neck aligned with your spine, looking down at the mat

- Engage your core to keep your torso stable as you 'swim'

KEY FOCUS POINTS:

- Keep movements fluid and graceful

- Resist the urge to lift your head, maintaining neck alignment

- Breathe steadily in rhythm with your 'strokes'

BENEFITS:

- Strengthens the back and core muscles

- Improves balance and coordination

- Enhances muscle control and proprioception

VARIATIONS AND ADAPTATIONS:

- If you have difficulty lifting both limbs simultaneously, lift one limb at a time

- Advanced users can speed up the 'swimming' action for more intensity

FREQUENCY AND DURATION: Perform for 30-60 seconds, 2-3 sets, twice a week

HALF-KNEELING WOOD CHOP

OBJECTIVE OF THE EXERCISE: To improve core rotational strength and stability from a challenging stance

DIFFICULTY LEVEL: Intermediate

EQUIPMENT NEEDED: A light dumbbell or resistance band

DESCRIPTION:

- Kneel with your right knee on the ground and left foot forward, left knee bent at 90 degrees
- Hold a dumbbell with both hands or the end of a resistance band anchored to your right
- Lift the weight or pull the band diagonally across your body to the upper left, rotating your torso
- Slowly return to the start, reversing the diagonal motion

KEY FOCUS POINTS:

- Keep your hips facing forward
- Use your core muscles to control the rotation
- Keep your arms extended, but not locked
- Maintain a steady breathing pattern

BENEFITS:

- Strengthens the core and upper body
- Improves balance in a less stable position
- Encourages rotational mobility and coordination

VARIATIONS AND ADAPTATIONS:

- Use a resistance band with less tension or no weight for an easier variation
- To increase the challenge, use a heavier weight or more resistant band

FREQUENCY AND DURATION: Perform 8-10 repetitions on each side, 2 sets, twice a week

DYNAMIC PLANK SHIFTS

OBJECTIVE OF THE EXERCISE: To build core strength and stability through dynamic movement in a plank position

DIFFICULTY LEVEL: Intermediate

EQUIPMENT NEEDED: Exercise mat

DESCRIPTION:

- Begin in a forearm plank position, ensuring your body forms a straight line from shoulders to heels
- Engage your core muscles, then slowly shift your weight forward as if trying to touch the wall in front of you with your nose

- Shift your weight back to the starting position

- Keep your movements small and controlled

KEY FOCUS POINTS:

- Ensure your hips and shoulders stay level throughout the exercise

- Avoid sagging or hiking your hips

- Keep your neck neutral and gaze down

BENEFITS:

- Improves dynamic core stability

- Enhances shoulder and arm strength

- Promotes endurance and muscular control

VARIATIONS AND ADAPTATIONS:

- For an easier variation, perform the plank with your knees on the ground

- To increase difficulty, perform the shifts on your hands instead of your forearms

FREQUENCY AND DURATION: Hold the plank for 20-30 seconds while performing shifts, 2-3 sets, every other day

RESISTANCE BAND TORSO TWISTS

OBJECTIVE OF THE EXERCISE: To enhance trunk rotational strength and stability using resistance

DIFFICULTY LEVEL: Intermediate

EQUIPMENT NEEDED: Resistance band

DESCRIPTION:

- Secure a resistance band at chest height

- Stand with your side to the anchor point, feet hip-width apart, holding the band with both hands in front of you

- With arms extended, rotate your torso away from the anchor point, keeping your hips facing forward

- Slowly return to the start position

KEY FOCUS POINTS:

- Engage your core throughout the twist

- Keep your arms extended but not locked

- Rotate only as far as comfortable without straining

BENEFITS:

- Strengthens core and oblique muscles

- Encourages control and stability during rotational movements

- Promotes shoulder mobility

VARIATIONS AND ADAPTATIONS:

- For beginners, reduce band tension or perform the twist without a band

- For added difficulty, increase band resistance or perform a squat simultaneously with the twist

FREQUENCY AND DURATION: Perform 10-12 twists on each side, 2 sets, three times a week

BALANCE BALL BRIDGE

OBJECTIVE OF THE EXERCISE: To enhance core stability and hip strength through a bridging motion on an unstable surface

DIFFICULTY LEVEL: Intermediate

EQUIPMENT NEEDED: Stability ball

DESCRIPTION:

- Lie on your back with your feet on top of a stability ball, knees bent, and arms at your sides for support

- Engage your core and lift your hips up into a bridge position

- Hold this position, ensuring that your body forms a straight line from shoulders to knees

- Gently roll the ball in towards your buttocks and then back out to the starting position

KEY FOCUS POINTS:

- Keep your movements controlled and steady

- Use your arms for stabilization but focus on using your core and hips for the movement

- Maintain even breathing

BENEFITS:

- Strengthens the glutes and core muscles

- Improves balance and stability

- Enhances control over an unstable surface

VARIATIONS AND ADAPTATIONS:

- To make it easier, perform the bridge with feet on the ground

- To increase difficulty, perform with one leg lifted while keeping the other on the ball

FREQUENCY AND DURATION: Perform 8-10 repetitions, 2-3 sets, twice a week

Chapter 5: Lower Body Workouts for Stability

Ankle and foot strength are critical components for balance and stability, as they form the base of our bodily structure. A strong foundation here aids in better distribution of weight and more adept movement, reducing the likelihood of falls and enhancing confidence in daily activities. The exercises in this series are designed to fortify those areas, improve proprioception—the body's ability to sense movement, action, and location—and support overall lower body strength. For seniors, focusing on these areas can profoundly impact their quality of life. From simple stretches to strengthening movements, these exercises are tailored for various fitness levels and can be performed safely and effectively at home.

Toe Taps

OBJECTIVE OF THE EXERCISE: To improve the control and range of motion in the ankle joints.

DIFFICULTY LEVEL: Beginner

EQUIPMENT NEEDED: None.

DESCRIPTION:

- Sit comfortably with your back straight and feet flat on the floor.
- Tap your toes on the ground while keeping your heel in a fixed place.
- Lift the toes as high as possible before returning them to the floor.
- Perform the exercise with a steady and controlled rhythm, ensuring movement comes from your ankles.

KEY FOCUS POINTS:

- Keep your movements slow and controlled.
- Maintain proper posture throughout the exercise.
- Focus on the up and down movement of your toes, avoiding any side-to-side motion.

BENEFITS:

- Increases ankle mobility and flexibility.
- Helps in preventing stiffness and improving circulation to the feet.
- Can lead to better balance and gait when walking.

VARIATIONS AND ADAPTATIONS:

- For variation, try tapping the feet alternately or to a rhythm in music.
- If sitting is uncomfortable, perform this exercise while standing and holding onto a stable surface for support.

FREQUENCY AND DURATION: 10 taps with each foot, 2-3 sets once a day.

Heel Raises

OBJECTIVE OF THE EXERCISE: To strengthen the calf muscles and the stability of the ankle.

"

Difficulty Level: Beginner to Intermediate

Equipment Needed: None or a stable surface for balance support.

Description:

- Stand upright with your feet hip-width apart.
- Gradually lift your heels off the ground, rising onto your toes.
- Hold the position briefly then slowly lower your heels back to the ground.
- Keep your core engaged and use a wall or chair for support if needed.

Key Focus Points:

- Focus on lifting your heels evenly.
- Engage your calf muscles fully during the lift.
- Make sure to rise and lower your heels smoothly without jerking.

Benefits:

- Strengthens the calf muscles and ankle joints.
- Improves balance and aid in activities such as climbing stairs or walking on uneven surfaces.

Variations and Adaptations:

- To increase difficulty, perform the exercise on one leg at a time.
- If balancing is challenging, perform the exercise seated with your weight slightly forwarded, lifting heels off the ground.

Frequency and Duration: Do 10-15 raises, repeat for 2-3 sets daily.

ANKLE CIRCLES

Objective of the Exercise: To enhance ankle flexibility and joint mobility.

Difficulty Level: Beginner

Equipment Needed: A chair for support if needed.

Description:

- Sitting down or standing, lift one foot off the ground.
- Rotate your foot to draw circles in the air with your toes.
- Perform clockwise circles, then switch to counterclockwise.
- Switch feet and repeat the exercise.

Key Focus Points:

- Keep the circles smooth and even.
- Perform circles without moving your leg or hip.
- If standing, ensure you are balanced and stable on the supporting leg.

Benefits:

- Promotes ankle flexibility and mobility.

- Helps reduce the risk of ankle sprains and strains by keeping joints lubricated.

VARIATIONS AND ADAPTATIONS:

- Perform seated for more stability.
- Adjust the size of your circles to increase or decrease difficulty.

FREQUENCY AND DURATION: Perform 10 circles in each direction for both ankles, 1-2 sets daily.

TOE SPREAD AND SQUEEZE

OBJECTIVE OF THE EXERCISE: To improve toe flexibility and strengthen the small muscles in the feet.

DIFFICULTY LEVEL: Beginner

EQUIPMENT NEEDED: None or a small, squeezable object.

DESCRIPTION:

- Sitting with your feet flat on the ground, spread your toes as far apart as possible.
- Hold the spread for a few seconds, then squeeze your toes together.
- If possible, place a small, soft object between your toes and practice squeezing it.

KEY FOCUS POINTS:

- Ensure you spread and squeeze your toes without straining.
- Keep your feet flat on the floor during the exercise.
- Maintain an upright posture throughout.

BENEFITS:

- Enhances toe dexterity and flexibility.
- Strengthens foot muscles contributing to overall stability.

VARIATIONS AND ADAPTATIONS:

- Utilize toe separators as a variation to increase stretch.
- Practice without an object for a less intensive version of the exercise.

FREQUENCY AND DURATION: Do 10 repetitions for each foot, complete 2-3 sets daily.

MARBLE PICKUPS

OBJECTIVE OF THE EXERCISE: To improve toe strength and precision of foot movements.

DIFFICULTY LEVEL: Intermediate

EQUIPMENT NEEDED: A bowl and several small objects such as marbles or pebbles.

DESCRIPTION:

- Place a bowl of small objects in front of you while seated.
- Using only your toes, pick up an object and transfer it to a different spot.
- Repeat the movement with each toe, trying to use only the toe muscles without assistance from your hands or legs.

KEY FOCUS POINTS:

- Use a gentle grip on the objects.
- Focus on isolating the movement to your toes.
- Remain seated to ensure safety while performing the exercise.

BENEFITS:

- Increases toe strength and control.
- Enhances the fine motor skills of the feet, contributing to better balance and stability when walking.

VARIATIONS AND ADAPTATIONS:

- For a more straightforward adaptation, use larger objects that are easier to grasp.
- To increase difficulty, use smaller and rounder objects like marbles.

FREQUENCY AND DURATION: Pick up and transfer 10 small objects, completing 2-3 sets with each foot daily.

MARBLE PICKUP

OBJECTIVE OF THE EXERCISE: To improve toe strength and coordination.

DIFFICULTY LEVEL: Beginner

EQUIPMENT NEEDED: A small bowl and marbles or similar small objects

DESCRIPTION:

- Sit in a chair with your feet flat on the floor and a bowl of marbles in front of you.
- Use your toes to pick up a marble and transfer it into an empty bowl beside the original.
- Continue to transfer marbles, one at a time, focusing on using only your toes.

KEY FOCUS POINTS:

- Ensure you're grasping the marbles firmly with your toes.
- Try to use different parts of the foot for added variety in the workout.
- Keep your back straight and avoid leaning too much into the movement.

BENEFITS:

- Strengthens the muscles in the toes and feet.
- Enhances toe grip and overall foot coordination, vital for maintaining balance when walking on uneven surfaces.

VARIATIONS AND ADAPTATIONS:

- Place the bowls at varying distances to adjust the difficulty level.
- If picking up marbles is too challenging, start with larger objects and progress to smaller ones.

FREQUENCY AND DURATION: Complete the transfer of 10-15 marbles, then repeat with the other foot, once a day.

OBJECTIVE OF THE EXERCISE: To improve ankle strength and mobility throughout its full range of motion.

DIFFICULTY LEVEL: Beginner

EQUIPMENT NEEDED: None

DESCRIPTION:

- Sit in a chair or on a bed with one leg extended straight out.
- Point your toe and "draw" each letter of the alphabet in the air with your big toe, moving only at the ankle.
- Keep your movements deliberate, ensuring full extension throughout the entire range of motion.

KEY FOCUS POINTS:

- Focus on creating clear and large letters.
- Keep your leg and upper body as still as possible.
- Proceed from letter A to Z with controlled, fluid movements.

BENEFITS:

- Increases ankle mobility and flexibility.
- Encourages fine motor control in the feet and lower leg muscles.
- Helps with coordination and proprioception, which are essential for balance.

VARIATIONS AND ADAPTATIONS:

- To add a challenge, perform the alphabet with your eyes closed to improve proprioception.
- If an entire alphabet is too demanding, start with just a few letters and build up over time.

FREQUENCY AND DURATION: Complete one full alphabet with each foot, once a day.

5.2 KNEE-STRENGTHENING AND STABILITY ROUTINES

Knee strength and stability are cornerstones of confident mobility for seniors, laying the groundwork for a vibrant, active lifestyle. The exercises I'm about to detail are thoughtfully designed to bolster the muscles surrounding the knee, enhancing support and movement control. We will focus on gentle yet effective routines that accommodate a range of fitness levels, all with the overarching aim to improve your quality of life. Let's embark on this journey together, nurturing the ability to perform tasks with greater ease and assurance.

OBJECTIVE OF THE EXERCISE: To strengthen the quadriceps and glutes, enhance knee stability, and practice the movement used in everyday living.

DIFFICULTY LEVEL: Beginner

EQUIPMENT NEEDED: A sturdy chair without wheels.

DESCRIPTION:

- Begin seated at the edge of the chair, feet planted firmly on the floor and hip-width apart
- Place your hands on your thighs for support
- Lean slightly forward and stand up slowly, using your leg muscles rather than your hands
- Gently lower yourself back into the seated position, controlling the motion without plopping down.

KEY FOCUS POINTS:

- Maintain even weight distribution between both feet
- Keep your chest raised and back straight throughout the movement
- Engage your core for stability
- Breathe out as you stand and breathe in as you sit back down.

BENEFITS:

- Improves muscle strength in legs and core
- Boosts functional movement for daily tasks like getting out of a chair
- Aids in joint health by promoting smooth motion.

VARIATIONS AND ADAPTATIONS:

- To add difficulty, cross arms over the chest or extend them forward instead of using thigh support
- For those with less strength, use your hands lightly for assistance on your thighs or the chair.

FREQUENCY AND DURATION: Perform 8-10 repetitions, twice a day.

KNEE EXTENSIONS

OBJECTIVE OF THE EXERCISE: To increase strength in the quadriceps muscles at the front of the thigh, which are crucial for knee stability and walking.

DIFFICULTY LEVEL: Beginner

EQUIPMENT NEEDED: A sturdy chair without wheels.

DESCRIPTION:

- Sit in the chair with your back straight and feet flat on the floor
- Extend one leg out in front of you until it is parallel to the floor
- Hold the position for a second, then slowly lower the foot back down to the floor
- Ensure movements are controlled and smooth.

KEY FOCUS POINTS:

- Focus on engaging your thigh muscles
- Keep the extended leg straight but avoid locking the knee
- Perform the extension slowly to maximize muscle engagement

- Keep your back against the chair.

BENEFITS:

- Strengthens the quadriceps
- Enhances knee joint stability for better balance and walking efficiency.

VARIATIONS AND ADAPTATIONS:

- Perform the exercise with a light ankle weight for increased resistance
- If fully extending the leg is too challenging, partially extend until strength improves.

FREQUENCY AND DURATION: Perform 10 repetitions on each leg, twice a day.

STANDING HAMSTRING CURLS

OBJECTIVE OF THE EXERCISE: To strengthen the hamstring muscles behind the thigh, important for walking and bending the knee.

DIFFICULTY LEVEL: Beginner to Intermediate

EQUIPMENT NEEDED: A sturdy chair or countertop for balance.

DESCRIPTION:

- Stand with your support in front of you, holding it for balance
- Keeping your thighs aligned, bend one knee to lift the heel toward your buttocks
- Hold the position briefly, then slowly lower the foot back to the floor
- Alternate legs after completing a set.

KEY FOCUS POINTS:

- Keep your supporting knee slightly bent
- Avoid swinging the leg or using momentum
- Keep your hips level and core engaged
- The movement should be smooth and controlled.

BENEFITS:

- Builds hamstring strength which complements the quadriceps
- Helps with movements such as climbing stairs and standing from a seated position.

VARIATIONS AND ADAPTATIONS:

- To increase difficulty, add an ankle weight
- For those with less leg strength, perform the motion without raising the heel as high.

FREQUENCY AND DURATION: Perform 8-12 repetitions on each leg, once a day.

SIDE-LYING LEG LIFTS

OBJECTIVE OF THE EXERCISE: To strengthen the hip abductor muscles, which support the knee by stabilizing the hip during walking.

DIFFICULTY LEVEL: Beginner

EQUIPMENT NEEDED: Exercise mat or a folded blanket for comfort.

DESCRIPTION:

- Lie on one side with your legs straight, propping your head up with your hand or resting it on your arm
- Lift the top leg upward, keeping it straight and aligned with your body
- Pause at the top, then lower it back down with control
- Repeat on the other side after completing a set.

KEY FOCUS POINTS:

- Keep your core engaged for added stability
- Avoid rolling your hips forward or back
- The lifted leg should be kept in line with the body, not forward or backward
- Movements should be slow and deliberate.

BENEFITS:

- Strengthens the side hip muscles for better balance and lateral stability
- Reduces pressure on the knees by providing stronger hip support.

VARIATIONS AND ADAPTATIONS:

- For a variation, point your toe slightly down to target the muscles more effectively
- If lying down is uncomfortable, perform standing leg lifts while holding onto a support.

FREQUENCY AND DURATION: Perform 10-15 repetitions on each side, once a day.

CALF RAISES

OBJECTIVE OF THE EXERCISE: To strengthen the calf muscles, which help with propulsion during walking and provide stability to the ankles and knees.

DIFFICULTY LEVEL: Beginner

EQUIPMENT NEEDED: A sturdy chair or countertop for balance.

DESCRIPTION:

- Stand with your feet hip-width apart, holding onto the support in front of you
- Rise onto your toes, lifting your heels off the ground
- Hold for a second at the top, then lower down slowly to the starting position.

KEY FOCUS POINTS:

- Keep the rise and descent controlled
- Distribute your weight evenly across the balls of both feet
- Engage your core for better balance
- Breathe out as you rise and in as you lower.

BENEFITS:

- Improves calf muscle strength for push-off during walking or climbing steps

- Supports ankle stability to reduce stress on knees

- Enhances overall balance when stationary or moving.

VARIATIONS AND ADAPTATIONS:

- To increase difficulty, perform the calf raise without holding onto a support for balance

- If full raises are too challenging, lift the heels only as high as comfortable.

FREQUENCY AND DURATION: Perform 10-15 repetitions, twice a day.

SITTING TO STANDING

OBJECTIVE OF THE EXERCISE: To strengthen the quadriceps and gluteal muscles, supporting knee stability and easing the transition from sitting to standing.

DIFFICULTY LEVEL: Beginner

EQUIPMENT NEEDED: A sturdy chair without wheels.

DESCRIPTION:

- Sit on the edge of the chair with feet flat and shoulder-width apart

- With arms crossed over the chest or stretched out in front for balance, lean slightly forward and push through your heels to stand up

- Pause at the top, then control your descent back into the sitting position.

KEY FOCUS POINTS:

- Keep your chest lifted and chin up as you stand

- Engage your core throughout the movement

- Ensure your knees do not go over your toes as you stand.

BENEFITS:

- Strengthens the muscles supporting the knee

- Enhances balance and functional mobility for daily activities.

VARIATIONS AND ADAPTATIONS:

- Add light hand weights to increase resistance

- Perform the movement more slowly for increased muscle engagement.

FREQUENCY AND DURATION: Perform 8-10 repetitions, once or twice a day.

LEG EXTENSIONS

OBJECTIVE OF THE EXERCISE: To strengthen the quadriceps and improve knee joint stability.

DIFFICULTY LEVEL: Beginner

EQUIPMENT NEEDED: A sturdy chair without wheels.

DESCRIPTION:

- Sit in a chair with back straight and arms resting on the chair or your lap

- Extend one leg straight out in front as much as possible, without locking the knee

- Flex your foot to engage the muscles, then lower back down with control.

KEY FOCUS POINTS:

- Keep your extended leg parallel to the floor

- Engage your core and maintain upright posture

- Point and flex the foot to engage different muscle groups.

BENEFITS:

- Improves quadriceps strength for better knee stability

- Enhances circulation in the lower extremities.

VARIATIONS AND ADAPTATIONS:

- Perform seated leg extensions with ankle weights for added resistance

- Alternate rapidly between legs for increased cardiovascular and muscular endurance.

FREQUENCY AND DURATION: Perform 10-15 repetitions for each leg, twice a day.

5.3 HIP MOBILITY AND STRENGTH WORKOUTS

The joys of movement often hinge on the fluidity and strength of one's hips. For seniors, maintaining hip mobility and stability is crucial as it plays a pivotal role in balance and the ability to perform everyday functions. Within this sub-chapter, we'll focus on exercises specifically designed to increase hip mobility and strength. These workouts are lovingly crafted to be practical, providing tangible benefits without overstraining tender joints. From gentle stretches to strength-building motions, each exercise is an opportunity to enhance your quality of life, giving you the freedom to move with confidence.

LYING HIP ROTATIONS

OBJECTIVE OF THE EXERCISE: To improve hip mobility and lubricate the hip joint.

DIFFICULTY LEVEL: Beginner

EQUIPMENT NEEDED: A mat or a flat, cushioned surface.

DESCRIPTION:

- Lie on your back with both knees bent and feet flat on the floor.

- Gently allow one knee to fall towards the floor, creating a rotating movement at the hip.

- Bring the knee back to the starting position and repeat on the other side.

- Keep the movements slow and controlled.

KEY FOCUS POINTS:

- Focus on keeping the opposite hip grounded during rotation.

- Ensure your back remains flat against the floor.
- Breathe deeply to encourage relaxation and aid in movement.

BENEFITS:

- Increases hip flexibility and range of motion.
- Encourages synovial fluid production, which can help ease hip stiffness.

VARIATIONS AND ADAPTATIONS:

- To modify, perform the exercise with one leg extended flat on the floor.
- Progress by holding the knee outward for longer before returning to start.

FREQUENCY AND DURATION: Complete 8 rotations per leg, once daily.

STANDING HIP ABDUCTION

OBJECTIVE OF THE EXERCISE: To strengthen the muscles on the outer thigh and hip for better stability.

DIFFICULTY LEVEL: Intermediate

EQUIPMENT NEEDED: A sturdy chair or countertop for support.

DESCRIPTION:

- Stand straight with your side facing the chair for support.
- Lift one leg out to the side, keeping the toe pointing forward.
- Slowly lower the leg back to starting position.
- Perform the movement without leaning to the opposite side.

KEY FOCUS POINTS:

- Keep your torso upright and avoid tipping to the side.
- Use the chair only for light support, not to hold your weight.
- Maintain a slight bend in the supporting leg for stability.

BENEFITS:

- Strengthens the hip abductors, which are critical for sidestepping and balance.
- Enhances overall leg coordination and muscular endurance.

VARIATIONS AND ADAPTATIONS:

- For a greater challenge, add ankle weights.
- To make it easier, limit the height of the leg lift.

FREQUENCY AND DURATION: Do 10-15 lifts per leg, two sets each, every other day.

HIP EXTENSION IN PRONE POSITION

OBJECTIVE OF THE EXERCISE: To enhance strength in the glutes and hamstrings, contributing to hip stability.

DIFFICULTY LEVEL: Beginner

EQUIPMENT NEEDED: A mat or a firm, padded surface.

DESCRIPTION:

- Lie face down with your head resting on your folded arms.
- Keeping one leg straight, lift it slowly off the ground, then lower it back down.
- Alternate with the other leg, ensuring movements are slow and controlled.

KEY FOCUS POINTS:

- Focus on using the glutes and hamstrings to lift the leg.
- Keep the hips and pelvis in contact with the ground.
- Avoid arching the lower back during the lift.

BENEFITS:

- Improves the strength of posterior chain muscles, essential for upright posture.
- Aids in the prevention of lower back pain by supporting proper alignment.

VARIATIONS AND ADAPTATIONS:

- To reduce intensity, perform a small range of motion lift.
- Increase difficulty by holding the leg up for a longer duration before releasing.

FREQUENCY AND DURATION: Aim for 8-12 lifts per leg, completing one set daily.

BRIDGE WITH HIP ADDUCTION

OBJECTIVE OF THE EXERCISE: To strengthen the glutes and inner thigh muscles, contributing to pelvic stability.

DIFFICULTY LEVEL: Intermediate

EQUIPMENT NEEDED: A mat and a small, soft ball or pillow.

DESCRIPTION:

- Lie on your back, knees bent, and feet flat on the floor, with a ball or pillow between your knees.
- Press your hips upward into a bridge while squeezing the ball.
- Hold for a few seconds, then slowly lower back to the floor.

KEY FOCUS POINTS:

- Ensure the lift comes from your hips and not the lower back.
- Keep your feet parallel and arms flat on the floor for support.
- Squeeze the ball consistently throughout the lift.

BENEFITS:

- Increases strength in the glutes and inner thighs.
- Promotes stability of the pelvic girdle, crucial for balance and walking.

VARIATIONS AND ADAPTATIONS:

- Remove the ball for a simpler bridge variation.

- Progress by holding the bridge position longer or adding a resistance band above the knees.

FREQUENCY AND DURATION: Perform 10-12 repetitions, two sets, three times a week.

SUPINE HIP ROTATION STRETCH

OBJECTIVE OF THE EXERCISE: To improve hip flexibility and encourage rotational mobility.

DIFFICULTY LEVEL: Beginner

EQUIPMENT NEEDED: A mat.

DESCRIPTION:

- Lie on your back, both knees bent and feet flat on the floor.
- Drop both knees to one side, keeping your shoulders on the floor, and hold the stretch.
- Bring knees back to center and repeat on the opposite side.

KEY FOCUS POINTS:

- Keep your upper body flat on the floor.
- Breathe deeply to enhance the stretch.
- Only stretch to the point of mild tension, not pain.

BENEFITS:

- Promotes flexibility in the lower back and hip rotators.
- Assists in reducing tightness and discomfort in the hips.

VARIATIONS AND ADAPTATIONS:

- For a gentler stretch, keep your feet further apart before rotating the knees.
- Advance the stretch by placing the ankle of one leg over the knee of the other before rotating.

FREQUENCY AND DURATION: Hold each stretch for 20-30 seconds, repeating two times on each side, once a day.

SIDE-LYING LEG RAISES

OBJECTIVE OF THE EXERCISE: To improve hip abductor strength, which supports lateral movement and stability.

DIFFICULTY LEVEL: Beginner

EQUIPMENT NEEDED: A mat or soft surface.

DESCRIPTION:

- Lie down on your side with your legs extended and your body in a straight line
- Rest your head on the lower arm, and place the top hand on the floor in front of you for stability
- Slowly lift the top leg as high as comfortable, then lower it back down with control
- Keep the leg straight and the movements smooth.

KEY FOCUS POINTS:

- Maintain a straight alignment from head to toe

- Focus on lifting the leg using the hip muscles, not momentum

- Breathe evenly throughout the exercise.

BENEFITS:

- Strengthens the hip abductors, which can reduce the likelihood of sideways falls

- Supports the hips in activities such as getting out of bed or stepping sideways.

VARIATIONS AND ADAPTATIONS:

- If lifting the leg becomes easy, add ankle weights for resistance

- For those with back issues, bend the bottom leg for additional support.

FREQUENCY AND DURATION: Perform 10-15 lifts on each side, once daily.

HIP CIRCLES

OBJECTIVE OF THE EXERCISE: To increase hip joint mobility and promote fluid movement in the pelvic area.

DIFFICULTY LEVEL: Beginner

EQUIPMENT NEEDED: None.

DESCRIPTION:

- Stand behind a chair, resting your hands on the backrest for support

- Shift your weight slightly to one foot

- Lift the opposite leg and begin to rotate the hip in circular motions

- Make 5 circles clockwise, then 5 counterclockwise

- Repeat with the other leg.

KEY FOCUS POINTS:

- Keep the standing leg slightly bent

- Make the circles as large as is comfortable without losing balance

- Use the chair for support but aim to engage the hip muscles.

BENEFITS:

- Improves hip flexibility and joint health, which is beneficial for walking and preventing stiffness

- Encourages better circulation in the lower extremities.

VARIATIONS AND ADAPTATIONS:

- For a greater challenge, perform the circles without holding onto the chair

- To modify, reduce the size of the circles if experiencing any discomfort.

FREQUENCY AND DURATION: Do 2-3 sets per leg, once daily.

Chapter 6: Upper Body Exercises for Postural Support

In this segment of our journey to enhance upper body strength and support, we'll focus on movements that fortify the shoulders and neck. These regions are pivotal for good posture and balance, often overlooked as we age. The exercises I'll introduce are specifically designed to maintain and improve the stability and functionality of these areas, helping you continue to perform daily activities with greater ease and confidence.

Shoulder Circle Warm-Up

Objective of the Exercise: To mobilize the shoulder joints and prepare the muscles for more intensive exercises.

Difficulty Level: Beginner

Equipment Needed: None

Description:

- Begin by standing or sitting upright with your arms relaxed at your sides
- Slowly roll your shoulders in a forward circular motion, starting with small circles and gradually increasing the size
- After completing the forward circles, change direction and perform the motion backwards
- Focus on smooth, controlled movements throughout the exercise.

Key Focus Points:

- Pay attention to any tension or discomfort in the shoulder area
- Keep your neck still to isolate the shoulder movement
- Breathe rhythmically to maximize comfort and mobility.

Benefits:

- Promotes circulation and flexibility in the shoulder joints
- Can reduce stiffness and improve range of motion.

Variations and Adaptations:

- If mobility is limited, perform the exercise with one shoulder at a time
- For more intensity, add light hand weights.

Frequency and Duration: Perform the exercise for 1-2 minutes, two times a day.

Wall Angels

Objective of the Exercise: To strengthen the shoulder blades and improve postural alignment.

Difficulty Level: Intermediate

Equipment Needed: A flat wall

DESCRIPTION:

- Stand with your back flat against a wall, feet shoulder-width apart

- Place your arms against the wall with elbows bent at 90 degrees, like a goal post

- Gently slide your arms up the wall, keeping contact with the wall, until they are fully extended above your head

- Slowly return to the starting position.

KEY FOCUS POINTS:

- Maintain contact between your head, shoulder blades, and tailbone with the wall

- Keep your lower back from arching excessively

- Slide arms smoothly along the wall without jerking.

BENEFITS:

- Enhances shoulder mobility and postural support

- Strengthens upper back and shoulder muscles

- Encourages proper spinal alignment.

VARIATIONS AND ADAPTATIONS:

- To increase the challenge, step your feet forward away from the wall

- If full arm extension is difficult, move your arms up as far as comfortable without strain.

FREQUENCY AND DURATION: Perform 8-10 repetitions, once or twice a day.

NECK TILTS WITH RESISTANCE

OBJECTIVE OF THE EXERCISE: To strengthen the neck muscles and improve flexibility.

DIFFICULTY LEVEL: Beginner

EQUIPMENT NEEDED: None

DESCRIPTION:

- Sit or stand with good posture

- Place your right hand against the right side of your head

- Gently apply pressure with your hand while tilting your head to the left, resisting the movement with your neck muscles

- Hold for a few seconds, then relax and repeat on the other side.

KEY FOCUS POINTS:

- Keep your movements slow and controlled

- Avoid shrugging your shoulders as you tilt

- Use gentle pressure, never causing pain.

BENEFITS:

- Strengthens the neck muscles

- Reduces the risk of neck stiffness and pain

- Encourages better alignment of the head and neck.

VARIATIONS AND ADAPTATIONS:

- If you need less resistance, perform the tilt without hand pressure

- For more challenge, gradually increase the duration of the hold.

FREQUENCY AND DURATION: Hold each tilt for 3-5 seconds; perform 5 repetitions on each side, once a day.

OBJECTIVE OF THE EXERCISE: To improve upper back strength and prevent slumping shoulders.

DIFFICULTY LEVEL: Beginner

EQUIPMENT NEEDED: None

DESCRIPTION:

- Sit or stand with arms at your sides

- Pull your shoulder blades back and down, as if trying to squeeze a pencil between them

- Hold this squeeze for a few seconds, then relax and repeat.

KEY FOCUS POINTS:

- Focus on squeezing the shoulder blades together without raising your shoulders

- Avoid holding your breath during the exercise

- Relax your neck throughout the movement.

BENEFITS:

- Strengthens the muscles between the shoulder blades

- Improves posture

- Can alleviate tension in the upper back and neck.

VARIATIONS AND ADAPTATIONS:

- Perform the exercise seated with back support to ensure proper posture

- For added difficulty, hold the squeeze for a longer duration.

FREQUENCY AND DURATION: Perform 10-15 repetitions, two to three times per day.

OBJECTIVE OF THE EXERCISE: To strengthen deep cervical flexor muscles for neck stability.

DIFFICULTY LEVEL: Beginner

EQUIPMENT NEEDED: None

DESCRIPTION:

- Sit in a chair with your back straight and shoulders relaxed

- Gently tuck your chin towards your neck, creating a double chin

- Hold this position for 5 seconds before releasing.

KEY FOCUS POINTS:

- Keep your eyes level and head straight

- Do not nod your head down

- The motion should be controlled and small.

BENEFITS:

- Promotes better neck alignment

- Can relieve tension headaches related to poor posture

- Enhances neck stability.

VARIATIONS AND ADAPTATIONS:

- Instead of sitting, perform the exercise standing with your back against a wall for additional posture support

- Increase the hold time as the exercise becomes easier.

FREQUENCY AND DURATION: Repeat the exercise 10 times, up to three times a day.

ARM RAISES TO SHOULDER HEIGHT

OBJECTIVE OF THE EXERCISE: To increase shoulder mobility and strength.

DIFFICULTY LEVEL: Beginner

EQUIPMENT NEEDED: None

DESCRIPTION:

- Sit or stand with arms relaxed by your sides

- Slowly raise your arms straight in front of you to shoulder height

- Pause briefly, then lower back to the starting position.

KEY FOCUS POINTS:

- Keep your arms straight but not locked

- Avoid raising your shoulders towards your ears

- Breathe out as you lift your arms and inhale as you lower them.

BENEFITS:

- Improves shoulder strength and range of motion

- Aids in maintaining functional arm movement for daily tasks.

VARIATIONS AND ADAPTATIONS:

- For those with limited range of motion, raise the arms only as high as comfortable without strain

- Add light weights or resistance bands to increase the challenge as you progress.

FREQUENCY AND DURATION: Perform 8-12 repetitions, twice a day.

OBJECTIVE OF THE EXERCISE: To stretch the chest and shoulder muscles, promoting better posture.

DIFFICULTY LEVEL: Beginner

EQUIPMENT NEEDED: A corner of a room or a doorway

DESCRIPTION:

- Stand facing the corner of a room or a doorway
- Place your forearms against the two walls with elbows slightly below shoulder height
- Gently lean forward until you feel a stretch across your chest and shoulders.

KEY FOCUS POINTS:

- Keep your spine straight
- Do not let your lower back arch as you lean in
- Hold the stretch without bouncing.

BENEFITS:

- Stretches the chest and front shoulder muscles, which can become tight from poor posture
- Encourages more open, relaxed shoulders.

VARIATIONS AND ADAPTATIONS:

- If the stretch is too intense, simply move your elbows lower or step closer to the corner or doorway
- Those with greater flexibility can deepen the stretch by stepping further in.

FREQUENCY AND DURATION: Hold the stretch for 20-30 seconds, repeat 2-3 times, at least once daily.

6.2 ARM AND WRIST EXERCISES FOR BETTER SUPPORT

In this sub-chapter, we explore arm and wrist exercises specifically designed for seniors to bolster their upper body support system. The strength and flexibility of the arms and wrists are vital for a range of daily activities, from lifting groceries to steadying oneself against a rail. The exercises provided here are aimed at improving muscle tone, enhancing joint flexibility, and reinforcing overall wrist and arm stability. By regularly practicing these movements, seniors can expect to enjoy greater confidence in their physical abilities and a more robust support mechanism for their postural health.

OBJECTIVE OF THE EXERCISE: To improve wrist flexibility and range of motion.

DIFFICULTY LEVEL: Beginner

EQUIPMENT NEEDED: None.

DESCRIPTION:

- Extend your arms in front of you with elbows straight and palms facing down.

- Rotate your wrists slowly, drawing big circles with your fingertips, first clockwise, then counterclockwise.

- Start with gentle movements, gradually increasing the size of the circles as flexibility improves.

KEY FOCUS POINTS:

- Keep your shoulders relaxed and down.

- Focus on smooth, controlled wrist rotations without moving your arms.

- Gradually increase the motion range as your wrists warm up.

BENEFITS:

- Promotes blood circulation within the wrists.

- Enhances wrist mobility, which is essential for daily activities that require fine motor skills.

VARIATIONS AND ADAPTATIONS:

- Try performing the exercise with your hands in fists or with your palms facing up for variety.

- For an added challenge, hold a light weight in each hand while rotating.

FREQUENCY AND DURATION: Perform for 2 minutes, two times a day.

ELBOW FLEXION AND EXTENSION

OBJECTIVE OF THE EXERCISE: To strengthen the muscles in the upper arms and maintain elbow joint function.

DIFFICULTY LEVEL: Beginner

EQUIPMENT NEEDED: None.

DESCRIPTION:

- Sit or stand with your arms at your sides and elbows tucked in.

- Flex your elbows to bring your hands towards your shoulders, then extend to straighten the arms.

- Keep the movements slow and controlled.

KEY FOCUS POINTS:

- Ensure that you move only your forearms while keeping your upper arms still.

- Keep your wrists straight to avoid strain.

- Breathe in as you lift and exhale as you lower your hands.

BENEFITS:

- Strengthens the biceps and triceps.

- Aids in the performance of lifting and reaching tasks.

- Maintains elbow flexibility.

VARIATIONS AND ADAPTATIONS:

- To increase resistance, hold a water bottle or can in each hand.

- For those with limited mobility, perform the exercise one arm at a time.

Frequency and Duration: Perform 12 repetitions, twice a day.

FOREARM PLANK

Objective of the Exercise: To strengthen the shoulders, arms, and wrists while engaging the core for added stability.

Difficulty Level: Intermediate

Equipment Needed: A mat or soft surface.

Description:

- Begin on all fours with your forearms flat on the mat, elbows beneath shoulders.
- Step your feet back to form a straight line with your body, keeping your forearms and toes on the floor.
- Hold this position, ensuring your body doesn't sag or arch excessively.

Key Focus Points:

- Align your head with your spine and keep your gaze down to maintain neck alignment.
- Engage your core to support your back.
- Distribute your weight evenly across your forearms and toes.

Benefits:

- Builds strength and endurance in the upper body.
- Engages the core for better balance and overall stability.

Variations and Adaptations:

- To modify, hold the plank from the knees instead of the toes.
- Advanced individuals can alternate lifting each leg while holding the plank.

Frequency and Duration: Hold for 20 seconds, repeat 3 times, with a rest in between.

ARM RAISES TO SIDE AND FRONT

Objective of the Exercise: To increase shoulder mobility and strengthen the deltoid muscles.

Difficulty Level: Beginner

Equipment Needed: None.

Description:

- Stand with your feet hip-width apart, arms at your sides.
- With palms facing down, slowly raise your arms to the side up to shoulder height, then lower.
- Repeat the movement, raising arms to the front this time.

Key Focus Points:

- Keep your movements controlled and smooth.
- Avoid shrugging your shoulders as you raise your arms.
- Breathe out as you lift and inhale as you lower your arms.

BENEFITS:

- Enhances shoulder flexibility and range of motion.
- Strengthens muscles needed for activities involving lifting and reaching out.

VARIATIONS AND ADAPTATIONS:

- Try alternating between side and front raises in one motion.
- Include light hand weights for increased resistance as you progress.

FREQUENCY AND DURATION: Perform 10 side raises and 10 front raises, twice a day.

WRIST FLEXOR STRETCH

OBJECTIVE OF THE EXERCISE: To improve flexibility in the wrist flexors and prevent stiffness.

DIFFICULTY LEVEL: Beginner

EQUIPMENT NEEDED: None.

DESCRIPTION:

- Extend one arm straight out in front of you, palm up.
- Use the opposite hand to gently pull back on the fingers of the extended hand toward the body, feeling a stretch in the underside of the forearm.

KEY FOCUS POINTS:

- Keep the elbow of the extended arm straight throughout the stretch.
- Hold the stretch without causing pain.
- Breathe steadily as you hold the position.

BENEFITS:

- Facilitates ease of wrist movements.
- Reduces the potential for wrist strain from repetitive motions.

VARIATIONS AND ADAPTATIONS:

- For a different stretch, turn the palm down and gently press the fingers toward the body with the opposite hand.
- If the stretch is too intense, lessen the pull on the fingers.

FREQUENCY AND DURATION: Hold the stretch for 30 seconds on each wrist, repeat twice a day.

WALL PRESS

OBJECTIVE OF THE EXERCISE: To strengthen the arm and shoulder muscles and enhance postural support.

DIFFICULTY LEVEL: Beginner

EQUIPMENT NEEDED: A flat wall.

DESCRIPTION:

- Stand facing the wall at arm's length

- Place your palms flat against the wall at shoulder height and shoulder-width apart

- Keeping your body straight, bend your elbows to bring your body closer to the wall

- Press back out to the starting position.

KEY FOCUS POINTS:

- Keep elbows at a comfortable angle

- Ensure your body moves as one unit, without sagging or arching your back

- Maintain a neutral wrist position throughout the movement.

BENEFITS:

- Strengthens the entire arm and increases shoulder stability

- Encourages better posture by engaging the upper back muscles.

VARIATIONS AND ADAPTATIONS:

- For added difficulty, perform the push on a slight incline using a sturdy table

- To decrease difficulty, stand closer to the wall.

FREQUENCY AND DURATION: Perform 10 to 12 repetitions, two times per day.

WRIST CURLS

OBJECTIVE OF THE EXERCISE: To increase forearm strength and improve wrist flexibility.

DIFFICULTY LEVEL: Beginner

EQUIPMENT NEEDED: A light dumbbell or a water bottle.

DESCRIPTION:

- Sit in a chair with your forearm resting on your thigh

- Hold the dumbbell with your palm facing up

- Curl the weight towards your bicep, keeping your forearm on your thigh

- Lower the weight back down.

KEY FOCUS POINTS:

- Ensure the movement is slow and controlled

- Keep your wrist straight to avoid strain

- Focus on moving only your wrist, not your arm.

BENEFITS:

- Enhances grip strength, which is crucial for daily activities

- Improves wrist flexibility and joint health.

VARIATIONS AND ADAPTATIONS:

- If holding a weight is uncomfortable, try using a resistance band instead

- For those without equipment, practicing the motion with no weight still provides benefit.

FREQUENCY AND DURATION: Complete 8-10 repetitions with each wrist, once a day.

Integration is key for full-body balance and stability, and this chapter focuses on exercises that enrich upper body strength while simultaneously engaging core and balance. Tailored for seniors, these routines are designed to improve postural support and incorporate movements that enhance day-to-day functional skills. Within these exercises, we acknowledge the range of abilities and motivate our senior readers to embark on a journey toward more confident, strong, and steady movements.

BALLOON PRESS

OBJECTIVE OF THE EXERCISE: To enhance coordination and upper body strength with a focus on maintaining posture and balance.

DIFFICULTY LEVEL: Beginner

EQUIPMENT NEEDED: One inflated balloon.

DESCRIPTION:

- Stand with a slight bend in your knees, feet hip-width apart, and hold the balloon with both hands in front of your chest.
- Gently press the balloon between your palms, engaging your chest muscles while keeping a steady posture.
- Hold the press for three seconds, then release.
- Repeat the press while maintaining your balance and ensuring your posture remains upright.

KEY FOCUS POINTS:

- Keep your shoulders relaxed and down.
- Engage your core during the exercise to aid in stability.
- Focus on maintaining an even breathing pattern throughout.

BENEFITS:

- Strengthens the chest and arms while activating core muscles, helping to support an upright posture.
- Encourages full-body balance through the gentle resistance of the balloon.

VARIATIONS AND ADAPTATIONS:

- Perform sitting on a stability ball for added balance work.
- Adjust the balloon's size to modify the difficulty of the press.

FREQUENCY AND DURATION: Do 2 sets of 12 presses, resting for 1 minute between sets.

WALL ANGEL WINGS

OBJECTIVE OF THE EXERCISE: To strengthen shoulder and upper back muscles, and improve postural alignment.

DIFFICULTY LEVEL: Beginner to Intermediate

EQUIPMENT NEEDED: Flat wall

DESCRIPTION:

- Stand with your back against a wall, feet slightly away from the base.
- Press your arms, back of the head, and shoulder blades against the wall with elbows bent and palms forward.
- Slowly glide your arms upward, keeping contact with the wall, as if making snow angel wings.
- Return to the starting position and repeat.

KEY FOCUS POINTS:

- Keep your head, spine, and hips in alignment against the wall.
- Avoid arching your lower back by activating your core.
- If shoulder mobility is limited, only raise arms as high as comfortable.

BENEFITS:

- Encourages correct posture through strengthening the upper back and shoulders.
- Enhances flexibility in the shoulder joint and upper body.

VARIATIONS AND ADAPTATIONS:

- For a more advanced version, perform with a resistance band around your wrists.
- If standing is difficult, execute the exercise seated on a chair without wheels.

FREQUENCY AND DURATION: Complete 2 sets of 8-10 repetitions, resting for 1 minute between sets.

PRAYER POSE PULSING

OBJECTIVE OF THE EXERCISE: To strengthen the muscles of the hands, forearms, and shoulders, while maintaining balance.

DIFFICULTY LEVEL: Beginner

EQUIPMENT NEEDED: None

DESCRIPTION:

- Stand with feet shoulder-width apart, palms together in front of your chest in a prayer pose.
- Press your palms together firmly, then release slightly in a pulsing motion.
- Keep your elbows at the height of your wrists, and maintain even pressure for each pulse.

KEY FOCUS POINTS:

- Align your posture, ensuring your head is over your shoulders and hips.
- The core should be engaged to support balance.
- Keep your elbows level with your wrists, not dropping below.

BENEFITS:

- Strengthens the forearms and improves wrist and hand stability, aiding in daily tasks such as opening jars.
- Enhances focus and balance when performed standing.

VARIATIONS AND ADAPTATIONS:

- To vary, press your palms at different heights or sit in a chair with back support for less intensity.
- Pulse more slowly for a greater challenge.

FREQUENCY AND DURATION: Complete 3 sets of 15 pulses, resting for 30 seconds between sets.

BOOK BALANCE NECK STRETCH

OBJECTIVE OF THE EXERCISE: To stretch neck muscles and promote flexibility while focusing on balance.

DIFFICULTY LEVEL: Beginner

EQUIPMENT NEEDED: A lightweight book.

DESCRIPTION:

- Stand tall, feet hip-width apart, and place a lightweight book on top of your head.
- Gently tilt your head to one side, bringing ear toward shoulder without letting the book fall.
- Hold for 5 seconds, then return to the starting position and tilt your head to the other side.

KEY FOCUS POINTS:

- Maintain an upright posture with your eyes looking forward.
- Keep the book balanced, which will help stabilize your movement.
- Perform the stretches slowly and gently.

BENEFITS:

- Improves neck flexibility and range of motion.
- Encourages balance and focus as you work to keep the book in place.

VARIATIONS AND ADAPTATIONS:

- For an added challenge, perform this exercise standing on a balance pad.
- Remove the book and increase the range of motion for a deeper stretch as flexibility improves.

FREQUENCY AND DURATION: Hold each stretch for 5 seconds on each side, repeat 5 times per side.

SLOW MOTION PUNCHES

OBJECTIVE OF THE EXERCISE: To improve upper body strength, coordination, and reflexes without compromising balance.

DIFFICULTY LEVEL: Beginner

EQUIPMENT NEEDED: None

DESCRIPTION:

- Stand with feet hip-width apart, knees slightly bent.

- Extend one arm forward in a slow punching motion while rotating the torso, then smoothly retract it back to the starting position.
- Alternate between arms while maintaining an engaged core and balanced stance.

KEY FOCUS POINTS:

- Focus on a controlled and measured punching motion.
- Keep your breathing even and your movements coordinated with your breath.
- Rotate the torso slightly for full engagement.

BENEFITS:

- Strengthens arm and shoulder muscles, and torso rotation improves balance and coordination.
- Helps sharpen reflexes and cognitive function through focused, deliberate movements.

VARIATIONS AND ADAPTATIONS:

- Intensify the exercise by holding light hand weights.
- Slow the punches down further to enhance balance challenge.

FREQUENCY AND DURATION: Perform 10-15 punches with each arm, completing 2-3 sets in total.

TOWEL SHOULDER FLOSSING

OBJECTIVE OF THE EXERCISE: To improve shoulder mobility and flexibility as well as upper body strength.

DIFFICULTY LEVEL: Intermediate

EQUIPMENT NEEDED: A small towel.

DESCRIPTION:

- Hold the towel taut between both hands, hands a little wider than shoulder-width apart.
- Keeping your arms straight, raise them above your head and behind your back as far as comfortable before returning to the front.

KEY FOCUS POINTS:

- Keep a gentle bend in the knees to maintain balance.
- Engage the core to provide stability.
- Maintain a firm grip on the towel throughout the movement.

BENEFITS:

- Increases range of motion in the shoulders, which can alleviate stiffness and pain.
- Strengthens arms and improves posture.

VARIATIONS AND ADAPTATIONS:

- Widen or narrow the grip on the towel to adjust the stretch.
- Sit on a stability ball for added balance work.

FREQUENCY AND DURATION: Complete 2 sets of 10 repetitions, with a 30-second rest in between.

OBJECTIVE OF THE EXERCISE: To build strength in the arms and shoulders, while promoting core and lower body stability.

DIFFICULTY LEVEL: Intermediate

EQUIPMENT NEEDED: A sturdy chair without wheels.

DESCRIPTION:

- Sit on the chair, hands beside hips gripping the front edge of the seat.
- Move forward off the chair, lowering your body towards the ground by bending the elbows, then push back up.
- Maintain an upright posture and engage the core to keep balance.

KEY FOCUS POINTS:

- Eyes forward.
- Bend elbows to a 90-degree angle.
- Avoid straining the shoulders by keeping them down away from your ears.

BENEFITS:

- Strengthens triceps, a key muscle group for arm stability and function.
- Enhances balance as the lower body stabilizes while the upper body moves.

VARIATIONS AND ADAPTATIONS:

- Place a cushion or soft mat under your feet for added comfort.
- Adjust the depth of the dip for comfort and ability.

FREQUENCY AND DURATION: Perform 8-10 dips, aim for 2 sets with a minute rest between.

Chapter 7: Balance in Motion

Walking is as fundamental to our daily lives as breathing. Yet, as we grow older, this simple act can become a source of concern. For seniors, establishing strong walking techniques is essential for stability and preventing falls. By refining the way we walk, we cultivate a steadier gait and a more profound confidence in our ability to navigate the world around us.

When it comes to walking, stability starts well before the first step. It's an orchestration of muscle coordination, joint flexibility, and mental focus. Let's explore how each element plays a part and how we can bolster them together for a sturdier stride.

The Importance of a Stable Base

Imagine your body as a tower. Just like any well-built structure, a solid base is key. Pay particular attention to your feet. They should be shoulder-width apart, offering a stable and robust foundation. Shoes play a significant role too; choose ones that support your arch and cushion your step, providing a better command over your terrain.

Posture: The Pillar of Walking

Think of your posture as the central pillar of that towering structure. Hold your head high, aligning it with your spine, and keep your gaze forward. Dropping your sight line not only brings down your posture but also your balance. Shoulders should be relaxed but straight, roll them back slightly and let the confidence flow through your stance.

Engaging the Core for Control

Your core muscles are akin to the cables that steady a suspension bridge. They help in keeping that tower of yours from swaying. Lightly engage your abdomen while walking—not so tight that you can't breathe comfortably, but enough to feel a sense of control in your midsection. This subtle contraction supports your back and keeps your posture in check.

Step Mechanics

A balanced walk is defined by even, controlled steps. Lift your foot and step from heel to toe, rolling smoothly through the foot. Avoid exaggerated steps; they disrupt the fluidity of movement. When your foot descends, think of it as a gentle landing rather than a firm stamp. This reduces the impact on your joints and enhances balance.

Arm Movements: Adding Rhythm to Your Walk

Swinging your arms in a relaxed, opposite rhythm to your legs adds dynamism and balance to your walk. It's the natural counterbalance that streamlines your motion. Remember to keep your arms at a soft bend and resist clenching your fists—it's all about ease and flow.

Breathing: Powering Your Steps

Breathing may be instinctive, but there's an art to syncing it with your walk. Inhale deeply through your nose, filling your lungs and then exhale through your mouth. Rhythmic breathing not only oxygenates your muscles but also keeps you centered and attuned to your body's rhythm.

Navigating Varied Surfaces

Walking on different terrains trains your body to adapt and react. While it's crucial always to be aware of your environment, expect and accept that not all paths are smooth. When transitioning from one surface to another, slow down and grant yourself time to adjust to the new ground underfoot.

Pace and Progression

The beauty of walking lies in its natural progression. You start at your own pace, attuned to your body's signals. There's no need to rush; stability thrives in deliberation. Gradually increasing your pace as your stability improves is the essence of progress. Remember, walking is not a race—it's a journey towards maintaining freedom of movement.

The Art of Turning

Turning requires a dance between balance and movement. Pivot on your foot, stepping in the direction of the turn to avoid a sudden twist in your hips, which can throw off balance. Keep your head up and look towards your new direction; your body naturally follows your eyes. Treat turns as purposeful maneuvers, embracing the change in direction as much as the path ahead.

Staying Focused

Distractions can topple stability. Whether it be uneven sidewalks, bustling crowds, or simply the sights and sounds around us, maintain a gentle focus on your path. It's this mindful presence that ensures each step lands safely.

Using Aids for Added Stability

There's no shame in using walking aids; view them as tools in your stability toolkit. Walking sticks or canes can extend your base of support and provide tactile feedback from the ground. If you choose to use a walking aid, ensure it's the correct height and you're well-practiced in using it—it should be a seamless extension of your motion.

Weathering the Weather

Environmental conditions affect how we walk. Wet, icy conditions demand a wider base for greater stability. Take shorter steps and pay attention to warning signs of slippery paths. Earlier in the day or late afternoons are typically best for avoiding crowds and extreme weather, making for a more stabilized and enjoyable walk.

Confidence in Collabration

The human aspect of walking—an arm from a friend, the presence of a companion—can bolster our confidence and balance. Walk with family, friends, or join a walking group. The encouragement and companionship they provide are not just for the spirit but for the body's stability as well.

In practicing these techniques, patience is your ally. Each nuance in your walking routine is an investment in your stability. It's the gradual improvements, those small triumphs, that lead to an overall confidence in motion. Celebrate every step and remember that with each walk, you're not only moving forward in space but also towards a deepening independence and a richer, safer quality of life.

Walking is more than just a mode of transportation; it's a bridge to staying engaged in the world around us. As you incorporate these techniques into your daily walks, remember that balance is a dance of many small adjustments, and with each step, you're mastering the art. Embrace the journey with each stride, and as always, walk tall, walk proud.

7.2 Turning and Pivoting Safely

As we move through life, one constant is the need for safe and fluid motion. For seniors, certain movements can present challenges, and learning to execute these actions correctly is essential for maintaining balance and reducing the risk of falls. One such critical aspect of daily movement is turning and pivoting. These are actions we perform without a second thought when we're younger, but with age, it becomes crucial to turn our attention to the proper mechanics of these seemingly simple maneuvers.

Turning and pivoting require a complex blend of balance, coordination, and body awareness—skills that we understandably take for granted in our youth but may require relearning and refining as we grow older. To turn safely means to reorient the direction of your body without losing stability. Pivoting is similar but involves a rotation around a single fixed foot, often necessitating greater control and balance.

A key to turning and pivoting safely is to reduce the swiftness and sharpness of movements, thereby lowering the risk of dizziness or imbalance. It's not just about being cautious; it's about retraining your muscles and your mind to move in harmony. Let's explore how to turn this knowledge into practical action, ensuring these activities are performed effectively to support a life full of movement and independence.

Understanding Your Body's Signals

First and foremost, understand that your body communicates with you. If you feel unsteady or dizzy while turning or pivoting, it's a sign to slow down and be more deliberate with your motions. This feedback is invaluable as you practice new techniques to improve your balance.

Practical Steps for Safe Turns

When it comes to making turns, the goal is to execute them in a controlled and staged manner. Think of a ballet dancer performing a pirouette—not a rushed spin, but a precise, graceful motion. Here's how to turn safely:

Prepare by standing firmly with your feet hip-width apart. This stance gives you a stable base to start.

Focus on something at eye level in front of you. This fixed point, known as a visual anchor, helps maintain balance.

Initiate the turn by stepping out with one foot. The idea is not to twist your body abruptly but to take a controlled step in the direction of the turn.

Follow through with the other foot, completing the turn in small steps. Imagine you're stepping on stones across a stream, where careful placement of each foot is required.

Complete the turn by realigning your feet with your shoulders, readjusting as necessary to find your balance.

Perform these steps with intention and at a pace that feels comfortable for you. The slower execution not only minimizes the risk of falling, but also strengthens the neuromuscular pathways vital to balance.

Mastering Pivots with Precision

Pivoting, while more challenging, follows the same principles of control and focus. To pivot safely requires the ability to rotate your body around a stationary leg:

Starting from the same stable standing position, shift your weight to one leg. This leg will become your anchor.

Turn your head in the direction of the pivot, allowing your body to follow naturally while keeping your anchor leg firmly in place.

Lift your free foot slightly off the ground and rotate it in the same direction as your head, allowing the heel to lead and the toe to follow.

Allow your anchor leg to pivot on the ball of your foot, letting the heel come off the ground gently.

Complete the pivot by bringing your feet together again and reestablishing your balanced stance.

Try to maintain a consistent rhythm and flow through the movement, preventing jerky actions that could compromise balance. Pivot practice can significantly enhance stability and body awareness.

Strengthening Exercises for Confident Movement

Enhancing your ability to turn and pivot isn't just about the techniques. Strengthening the muscles that support these movements is equally important. Here are a few exercises to consider:

Leg lifts and holds to strengthen the thighs and improve balance.

Standing calf raises to build ankle stability.

Toe tapping while seated to increase blood flow and maintain flexibility in your feet and ankles.

Daily Life Integration

All these exercises and techniques should be integrated into your daily life. Make a conscious effort to practice controlled turns when navigating through rooms, or do calf raises while waiting for the kettle to boil. Embrace the dance of daily life with mindful pivots and turns as you transition from one task to the next.

While turning and pivoting are everyday movements, they play an outsized role in maintaining balance and safety. Whether it's repositioning yourself to face a loved one or changing course to admire a beautiful garden, how we maneuver in our space is key to our confidence and independence. By approaching these actions mindfully and with purpose, we ensure that each step—no matter how small—is safe, secure, and ultimately, freeing.

Embracing Change with Positivity

Adopt these techniques with a sense of adventure. Each new day is an opportunity to refine and rejoice in movement, to celebrate the extraordinary capacity of our bodies to learn and adapt at any age. Be patient with yourself as you incorporate these changes. Rejoice in the realization that turning and pivoting safely adds versatility to your motion and an extra layer of protection from falls.

Turning and pivoting are not just physical acts but are symbols of the dynamic lives you continue to lead. Each safe and stable twist or pivot is a triumph. It's about the joy in moving with confidence, the freedom to face any direction life may beckon, and the understanding that balance in all things is the cornerstone of a life well-lived. Let's keep moving, pivot gracefully through life's turns, and enjoy the balance and freedom it brings.

As we gently embrace the golden years, our bodies—and the way they move—start to tell a complex and beautiful story of a life well-lived. Within this narrative lies the vital theme of coordination, that harmonious conductor orchestrating the symphony of upper and lower body movements. Mastering this coordination not only enriches the melody of our daily lives but also fortifies the very essence of our balance and mobility. Imagine this: You're in the kitchen, reaching for a cup on a high shelf while steadying yourself on tip-toes. In that moment, a delicate dance unfolds between the stretching of your arms and the anchoring of your legs. This is the essence of upper and lower body coordination, a skill indispensable for preserving our independence and increasing our resilience against the unexpected.

But why is this coordination so crucial? It boils down to the reality of complex movements—those involving multiple muscle groups and joints across our bodies. From walking up a flight of stairs to engaging in a delightful round of gardening, these actions require a symphony of movement that grows less intuitive with age.

The Magic of Coordinated Movements

Movement coordination stems from more than just muscle; it's a holistic blend of nerves, muscles, and cognition—all of which need to be in fine fettle. Within these intertwined systems, our nerves fire off messages like lightning bolts across the grey skies of our nervous system, instructing muscles to contract, extend, and synchronize their efforts.

When we refine this coordination, we navigate our environments with more grace, lessen the load on our joints, and reduce the likelihood of injury. In terms of falls—a specter no one is keen to encounter—being adept at coordinating movements can be the difference between a catch and a tumble.

Moving Together: A How-To Guide

How do we foster this wondrous coordination? It starts with exercises that nurture the dialogue between our brains and limbs. We shall not leap headfirst into the deep end, but rather wade into the shallows, gradually deepening our capabilities.

Tandem Activities: Begin with movements easy to embrace, such as walking while moving your arms in a natural opposite rhythm. Think of it as a stroll in the park; your left foot steps forward as your right arm swings ahead. This is the baseline from which we build.

Synchronized Swimming on Land: Envision the grace of a synchronized swimmer and replicate it on terra firma. For instance, while standing, lift your right knee as you raise your left arm overhead—then alternate. These fluid movements intertwine the fates of your limbs, laying the groundwork for automatic responses in your daily life.

Mirror Games: Pair up with a friend or reflect your own movements in the mirror. Lift your leg as your partner does the same, and observe. Not only is this fun, but it also bolsters the connection between visual cues and physical response, essential for avoiding impediments in your path.

Dancing: The unspoken poetry of the dance is not merely for the spry and limber. Simple steps aligned with music strengthen neural pathways while fostering joy. Waltz through your living room, every step a chance to practice gentle turns and transitions.

Tai Chi: This ancient art, a ballet of the deliberate and mindful, hones the synchronization between upper and lower realms. Its measured movements are like flowing water—continuous and ever-adapting.

Strengthen. Then Coordinate.: Engage in strength exercises separately for upper and lower regions first. Once you gain confidence, combine these elements. A leg squat paired with an upward stretch, a calf raise while curling weights—marriages of movement that nurture coordination.

Safety Before Symmetry

As we cherish the joys of coordinated movement, let us not neglect the foundation upon which they rest— safety. Always ensure a secure environment, free from tripping hazards. Employ chairs or walls for support as you refine your prowess with these activities.

Adapting to Your Rhythm

Every body hums its own unique tune, so adapt exercises in tune with your individual rhythm. A step might be smaller, a reach less high, but the essence of the movement—the coordination—is what we seek to capture and develop.

The Ripple Effects of Coordination

Beyond the outright benefits to balance and stability, coordinated movements extend their grace to other facets of life. They can enhance cognitive function through the multi-tasking they demand, improve the heart's rhythm, and even lend depth to social interactions.

Remember to savor the pleasure found in the simplest of coordinated actions—buttoning a shirt, playing an instrument, or clasping the hands of a grandchild. Each feat is a testament to the seamless teamwork between your upper and lower halves.

Patience and Persistence: The Twin Pillars of Progress

The art of coordination is not a script written overnight. It's a narrative crafted over chapters, through the dedication of timeless patience and the resolve of unwavering persistence. Be kind to yourself as you traverse this path. Celebrate the smallest of victories, for they are but stepping stones to the grand triumph of your ongoing journey.

In Conclusion

As we integrate these practices into the fabric of our daily lives, we find that the true freedom lies not merely in the ability to stand tall, but in moving through life's myriad landscapes with an assured and harmonious stride. Here's to the wondrous possibilities that await, for just as every new dawn promises the light of day, so too does each step taken in coordination herald the dawning of renewed independence.

With each passing day, let us strive to weave the threads of upper and lower body movement into a tapestry rich with the hues of stability, confidence, and the bliss of unfettered motion. Together, guided by understanding and patience, we can waltz into a future where balance is not a fleeting note but the very melody of our existence.

Chapter 8: Advanced Balance Challenges

Multi-Directional Movements: The Gateway to Expanded Horizons

As we voyage further into the heart of balance mastery, let's embrace the wonder of multi-directional movements. These aren't just exercises; they're an exploration into the very poetry of motion, encompassing the myriad of ways we navigate the rich tapestry of life's landscape.

The very essence of multi-directional movements lies in their ability to simulate real-life scenarios. Whether it's reaching up to a high shelf, stepping carefully over a garden hose, or navigating through a crowded farmers market, our bodies are designed to move in more ways than merely forward and back. By incorporating side-to-side, rotational, and diagonal movements into our balance routines, we not only enhance our stability but also forge resilience against the unexpected.

Nowhere is the charm of the unexpected more evident than in a grandparent playing tag with a grandchild. The sudden shifts, the pivots, the agile side-steps—all these gestures require a harmony of balance that multi-directional training can provide. But why are these movements so beneficial, particularly for seniors seeking to enrich their quality of life?

The Benefits Unveiled

Let's look at the tapestry of benefits multi-directional training can provide. Firstly, it brings a holistic improvement to your proprioception—the body's awareness of itself in space. The more you train, the more adept your body becomes at adjusting to shifts in center of gravity, thus improving your reaction time. There's also the aspect of muscle engagement; these movements recruit various muscle groups, forming a cohesive unit that supports overall stability.

There's a particular beauty in how multi-directional movements train our minds as well as our bodies. Cognitive function receives a boost as the brain orchestrates the complex dance of muscles and balance. Yes, these exercises are a workout for your body's physical prowess and your brain's executive command.

Another key benefit is the break from monotony. Varied movements keep the mind engaged, reduce boredom, and increase the likelihood of sticking with your exercise routine. When exercises are enjoyable and challenging, your commitment naturally deepens—a crucial factor in maintaining a fitness regime.

Embracing the Freedom of Movement

At this point in our journey, it might feel daunting to embark on what seems like high-skill exercises. The truth is, you are more capable than you might believe. Each new step is a milestone in rediscovering your body's innate ability to move with grace and strength, akin to a dancer learning the steps to a new choreography.

As we begin, remember to honor your own pace. This isn't a race; it's about finding a personal rhythm, one where comfort and challenge coexist. With consistency and practice, your confidence will grow, making way for a new dimension of freedom.

Stepping into Action

Let's apply the theoretical knowledge to practical scenarios. Start with basic multi-directional steps, and as you grow more comfortable, infuse them with complexity.

Picture the ground as a clock: face forward—12 o'clock is straight ahead, 3 o'clock to your right, 6 o'clock behind you, and so forth. With this visualization, we can begin our adventure.

Forward and Sideways Steps: Imagine stepping onto 2 and then 10 o'clock positions, a fluid motion mimicking the natural stride but with a slight diagonal. This simple yet effective motion paves the way to maneuvering in more complex environments.

Backward Diagonal Steps: Once forward steps feel routine, try stepping back to 4 and 8 o'clock positions. Initially, use a chair or wall for support. Here, the backward motion engages different muscles and improves your ability to navigate spaces safely.

Rotational Steps: Rotate gently as if to step to 3 and 9 o'clock. The turning movement sharpens your ability to pivot—a skill that proves invaluable in avoiding obstacles.

Now, let's weave these steps together into fluid movements. Gradually eliminate the use of support as your confidence ascends.

Incorporating Movement Sequences

As your command of multi-directional steps solidifies, introduce sequences that mimic the natural flow of daily life. For instance, step to 2 o'clock, pivot to face 3 o'clock, and then step back towards 6 o'clock. Rehearse this dance, and you will start to notice an elegance to your maneuvers.

A delightful way to integrate these sequences is in tandem with chores or hobbies. Reach diagonally to water plants, or perform a gentle pivot while cooking to foster an environment where balance training is seamlessly merged with your everyday routines.

Propping Up the Challenge

To amplify the engagement, props can be advantageous. Use cones, pillows, or other markers to create a path requiring various directional steps. Weave through them, and you will be elated at how your agility improves—the key to navigating the unpredictability of the world outside your door.

Safety First: A Gentle Reminder

With progress comes the temptation to push boundaries. While commendable, never compromise safety for the sake of advancement. Always ensure a hazard-free area and have support close at hand. It's about embracing challenge, but with the wisdom to know your limits.

Concluding with a Reflection

Multi-directional movements are an invitation to defy the boundaries that age may impose upon us. They are an affirmation that our bodies, much like our spirits, need not be restrained by any one direction. It's about cultivating a belief—an article of faith in one's own strength and agility.

The underlying message is simple yet profound: life is a medley of directions, and moving through it with equilibrium and poise is not only possible, it's within reach. With every twist, turn, and step, you are painting your own masterpiece of movement that tells the story of a life lived fully and freely.

So, step forward—or sideways, or backwards—and reclaim the vast expanse of your world. A balanced life is a canvas awaiting your brush, and each direction you master is another stroke of vibrant color on the masterpiece that is your life's journey.

Enriching your balance exercises by incorporating props is an excellent way to challenge your body, engage your mind, and have a bit of fun along the way. These tools can provide support while simultaneously increasing the difficulty level of your workouts, making them an indispensable part of advanced balance training for seniors.

Using props effectively can transform the mundane into the extraordinary, as they add variety to your routines and can simulate real-life scenarios that improve your functionality in day-to-day activities. Whether you have cans of soup, a sturdy chair, or resistance bands, each prop has the potential to boost your balance capabilities.

Let's embark on a journey of exploration, delving into a few handy props and how they can work wonders for your balance and stability.

Stability Ball for Dynamic Sitting

Imagine a giant, inflatable ball that not only serves as a seat but also introduces an element of instability that your body must counteract to remain poised. This is the principle behind using a stability ball. Sitting on it requires constant micro-adjustments from your core muscles, promoting strength and balance without putting excessive strain on your joints.

Foam Pads and Balance Discs for Groundwork

When you step on a foam pad or a balance disc, the uneven surface forces your feet and ankles to work harder to maintain your equilibrium. By standing on these props, you can simulate the experience of walking on an uneven path, enhancing your ankle stability and reaction time. Progressing from two feet to one foot increases the challenge and benefits.

Resistance Bands for Muscular Endurance

Incorporating resistance bands into your balance exercises is like having a gym in a bag. These simple, elastic tools can add resistance to movements, engaging both your stabilizing muscles and the primary muscle groups. For example, standing on one leg while pulling a resistance band can help build hip and leg strength crucial for balance.

Wobble Boards for Coordination

Wobble boards are circular platforms with a domed bottom that require you to maintain your center of gravity over a constantly changing base of support. They are spectacular at improving proprioception – the body's ability to sense its position in space – and are particularly good at enhancing coordination and joint stability.

Hand Weights for Postural Alignment

Light hand weights can do more than just strengthen your muscles; they can also improve your balance by adding a load that your body must adapt to. Performing upper-body exercises while standing on one leg or walking can challenge your postural control and demand greater core activation.

Navigating the Props

Using props requires forethought and caution. It is essential to select them based on their suitability for your fitness level and balance proficiency. Always ensure that the prop is in good condition and placed on a non-slip surface to prevent accidents.

Stability Ball Exercises

Sit comfortably on a stability ball with your feet flat on the ground, shoulder-width apart. Aim to maintain an upright posture, engaging your core muscles to keep yourself steady. From this starting position, you can perform a variety of exercises:

Pelvic Tilts: Gently rock your pelvis forward and backward, engaging your abdominal muscles.

Arm Raises: With or without hand weights, alternate raising your arms to the front, side, and above your head.

Leg Lifts: Lift one foot off the ground at a time, maintaining balance as you do so.

Foam Pad and Balance Disc Exercises

Simply standing on a foam pad or balance disc can significantly enhance your balance. Try these exercises:

Standing Still: Begin by standing with both feet on the prop and hold for 30 seconds to a minute.

Weight Shifts: Shift your weight from one foot to the other, gradually trying to lift one foot off the prop entirely.

Squats: Perform squats while standing on the foam pad, ensuring your knees stay aligned over your feet.

Resistance Band Exercises

Resistance bands are versatile and can be used in seated or standing positions:

Seated Row: Sitting on a chair, place a resistance band around your feet. Hold the band with both hands and pull back, mimicking a rowing action.

One-Legged Band Pull: Stand on one leg, hold the band in both hands, and extend your arms forward, then pull back towards your chest.

Wobble Board Exercises

Start with the basics on the wobble board and progress from there:

Balance Hold: Stand on the wobble board with your feet spread evenly. Try to maintain your balance without letting the edges touch the ground.

Squats: After mastering the balance hold, try performing squats on the wobble board.

Hand Weight Exercises

Use light hand weights to improve your upper body strength while challenging your balance:

Walking in Place: As you march in place, perform bicep curls or shoulder presses.

One-Legged Stand: Stand on one leg and perform side raises or front raises with the weights.

Varying your balance exercises with props can turn a static routine into an engaging and effective workout. As you incorporate these tools into your balance training, remember that consistency is vital. Regular practice will improve your skill and confidence over time.

Safety is paramount, so always listen to your body's cues and don't hesitate to ask for assistance from a caregiver or fitness professional while trying new exercises with props.

In the world of balance and stability, props can be your steadfast allies. By integrating these tools into your regimen, you'll not only enhance your physical health but may also discover a newfound sense of freedom and enjoyment in your workouts. Here's to a balanced life, with every step assured and every movement full of grace.

The art of maintaining balance is, by nature, a dynamic challenge—one that requires not only steadiness but also the strength to navigate life's unexpected turns with grace and confidence. As we reach the latter years, the addition of light weights into our balance routines can be the golden thread that weaves strength and poise into the tapestry of our daily lives. This nuanced approach to balance training, with the careful use of light weights, holds the key to unlocking a newfound sense of control and vigor.

Imagine your body as a grand symphony, where each movement is a note and balance is the harmony. Light weights become the conductor's baton, instructing your muscles to play in perfect synchrony, creating a musical masterpiece of movement. As you incorporate these instruments into your routines, you are not merely exercising—you are orchestrating a symphony of stability.

The Philosophy Behind Weights in Balance Training

Weight training has been a cornerstone of exercise regimens for ages, celebrated for its capacity to build strength, endurance, and muscular definition. But when crafted with the needs of seniors in mind, it transcends the purely physical, becoming a means to elevate balance and poise to a level once thought beyond reach.

Apprehension might arise from the notion of integrating weights into balance exercises, especially with common misperceptions of weightlifting being reserved for the young or the Herculean. Let us dispel those myths at once. In the realm of balance for seniors, light weights serve not as a brutish force but as an ally—a subtle nudge that reminds your body of the strength it harbors within.

How Light Weights Enhance Balance

The crux of using light weights in balance exercises is not to bulk up but to fine-tune the body's proprioceptive abilities—the internal sense that tells you where your body is in space. With the gentle inclusion of weights, muscles must adapt and respond with greater precision, fostering improvements in coordination and postural alignment.

Moreover, the addition of resistance training stimulates bone density and joint health, fortifying the support system your balance so heavily relies upon. It is not merely about standing steady; it is about weaving resilience into the fabric of your muscles and bones.

The Practical Approach to Weighted Balance Training

Now, let us embark on the journey of incorporating light weights into our balance routines with a methodical and secure approach. Safety is paramount. Begin with the lightest weights—1 to 2 pounds can be sufficient. These weights can be hand-held dumbbells, ankle weights, or even everyday household items, such as cans of soup with equal weight, that rest comfortably in your hands.

The Rhythmic Start: Standing Tall with Weights

Begin your practice by standing with your feet shoulder-width apart, a weight in each hand, arms resting gently at your sides. Draw in a deep breath and as you exhale, intentionally ground yourself, feeling the floor beneath your feet, the air surrounding your frame, the weight in your hands as an extension of your own body's intention.

Lift the weights slowly with elbows bent, akin to the motion of starting a lawnmower, then gently lower them. With each lift and lower, engage your core—your abdominal muscles—feeling them support your every move. Your stance becomes not just a position but a statement of control.

Dynamic Balance Enhancement: The Weight Shift

One of the most practical exercises to include in your repertoire is the sideways weight transfer. Standing as before, hold a weight in your right hand. Shift your weight onto your left foot, lifting your right foot just a few inches off the ground. Pass the weight to your left hand while remaining balanced on your left foot. Then, return the weight to your right hand as you place your right foot down and shift weight onto it, lifting your left foot. Repeat this dance of balance, each transfer a deliberate and controlled movement.

Cognitive Engagement: The Upper-Lower Synchronization

Incorporating light weights does not solely enhance physical balance; it sharpens the mind. As you lift a weight with one hand, lift the opposite knee to meet it, then lower both in unison. This synchronization of limbs demands focus and reinforces the neural pathways that govern coordinated movement—a vital asset in maintaining balance.

Squats: The Foundation of Functional Strength

Squats are a powerful exercise for developing lower body strength, and the addition of light weights amplifies their impact. Holding weights at shoulder level, descend into a squat as though sitting back into a chair, then rise back up. Keep your back straight, and engage your core to protect your spine—a fortress safeguarding your balance.

The Balancing Act: Single-Leg Stance with Weights

An elevated challenge in balance training is the single-leg stance. Stand behind a sturdy chair, using it for support as needed. Lift one foot slightly off the ground, weight in hand on the same side, and hold. The other hand, with a weight, can stretch out for counterbalance. Swap sides after several seconds. Over time, reduce reliance on the chair, aiming for a freestanding display of balance.

Progress and Adaptation: The Weighted March

Take the classical marching in place and inject it with the challenge of weights. Lifting your knees high, alternate each leg, all while performing arm curls with the weights. This act unifies the body's strength with the mind's rhythm, a marriage of movement that epitomizes balanced strength.

Safety Considerations and Final Musings

While incorporating light weights offers a bounty of benefits, heed these words of caution: monitor your breath, avoid holding it, and always maintain a controlled motion. If discomfort arises, lower the weight or cease the movement. Listen to your body, responding to its dialogue with respect and kindness.

Throughout this journey, recall the importance of patience and perseverance. Building balance with the help of light weights is akin to cultivating a garden. It takes time, care, and consistent effort. The fruits of your labor will blossom, not overnight but over time, in a display of poise, resilience, and a triumphant stability that speaks of your dedication.

Harbor no doubt that the gentle introduction of light weights into your balance exercises paves the way for a vibrant form of stability, one that you will carry with pride down the corridors of life. With each lift, each shift, each measured step, you are etching into existence a newfound sense of freedom—a balance that once felt elusive but is now firmly within your grasp.

Chapter 9: Flexibility and Balance

Flexibility is the unsung hero of our daily movements, often overlooked but essential for a life rich with activity and ease. As we age, maintaining our flexibility becomes a cornerstone for balanced living. The following exercises are designed to gently stretch and lengthen muscle fibers, encourage proper joint function, and enhance the freedom of movement necessary for a vibrant life. These stretches will not only support your physical mobility but also contribute to a serene state of mind as you sync your breath with each motion, crafting a holistic approach to your well-being.

Toe and Heel Raises

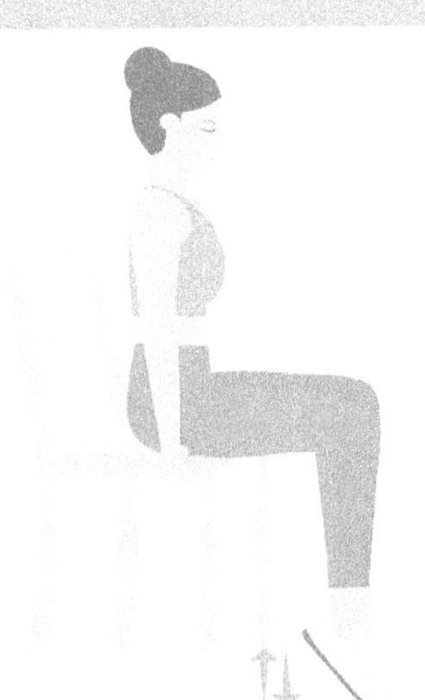

Objective of the Exercise: To increase the flexibility and range of motion in the ankle joint, improving circulation.

Difficulty Level: Beginner

Equipment Needed: None.

Description:

- Sit on a chair with your feet flat on the ground.
- Slowly lift your toes while keeping your heels on the ground, then lower your toes and lift your heels.
- The movement should be fluid and controlled, focusing on stretching the muscles in your lower legs.

Key Focus Points:

- Keep your back straight and avoid leaning too far forward or backward.
- Engage your core for stability.
- Focus on moving only your feet, keeping the rest of your body still.

Benefits:

- Improves flexion and extension in the ankles, promoting better balance.
- Encourages better circulation in lower extremities, which can reduce swelling and discomfort.

Variations and Adaptations:

- Perform this exercise seated or standing behind a chair for support if you want a bit more challenge.
- For those with reduced mobility, perform the raises one foot at a time.

Frequency and Duration: Perform 2 sets of 10 repetitions daily.

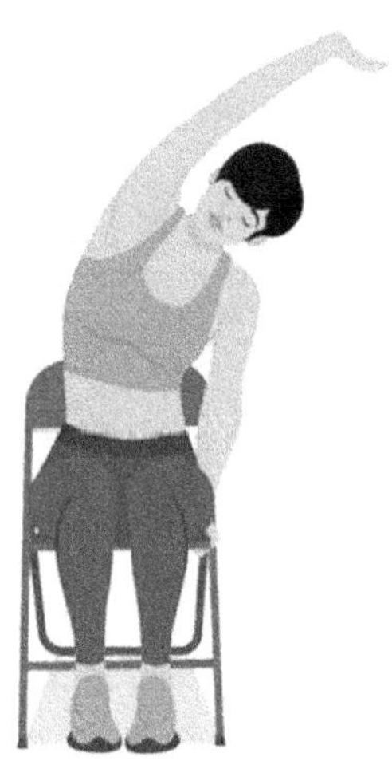

OBJECTIVE OF THE EXERCISE: To elongate the torso's muscles, increasing lateral flexibility and improving breathing capacity.

DIFFICULTY LEVEL: Beginner

EQUIPMENT NEEDED: A sturdy chair.

DESCRIPTION:

- Sit up straight in your chair without leaning on the backrest.
- Reach one arm overhead and bend to the opposite side, keeping your hips firmly in the chair.
- Hold the stretch for a few deep breaths, then return to the starting position and repeat on the other side.

KEY FOCUS POINTS:

- Ensure that your movements are smooth and steady.
- Do not strain or push too far; only stretch as much as is comfortable.
- Keep your buttocks on the chair to prevent tilting.

BENEFITS:

- Enhances elasticity of the oblique muscles.
- Aids in opening the rib cage for deeper breathing.
- Can alleviate stiffness in the upper body.

VARIATIONS AND ADAPTATIONS:

- Adapt the stretch by using a towel held in both hands to maintain arm alignment and encourage a deeper stretch.
- Reduce range of motion if experiencing pain or discomfort.

FREQUENCY AND DURATION: Hold the stretch for 20-30 seconds on each side, perform 1-2 times per day.

OBJECTIVE OF THE EXERCISE: To improve flexibility and range of motion in the wrists and forearms.

DIFFICULTY LEVEL: Beginner

EQUIPMENT NEEDED: None.

DESCRIPTION:

- Sit or stand with your arm extended at shoulder level.
- Flex your wrist downward, using the opposite hand to apply gentle pressure on the back of your hand.
- Then, extend your wrist upward, applying pressure to your fingers with the opposite hand.

KEY FOCUS POINTS:

- Keep your arm straight during the stretch.

- Do not force the wrist beyond its comfortable range of motion.

- Use the opposite hand to apply only gentle pressure.

BENEFITS:

- Increases wrist flexibility, which is beneficial for daily tasks like writing or cooking.

- Can help to alleviate wrist strain from repetitive activities.

VARIATIONS AND ADAPTATIONS:

- For a gentler stretch, perform without using the opposite hand for pressure.

- For a deeper stretch, increase the pressure slightly but always within a pain-free range.

FREQUENCY AND DURATION: Hold each stretch for 15-20 seconds, repeating 2-3 times per wrist, once daily.

NECK CIRCLES

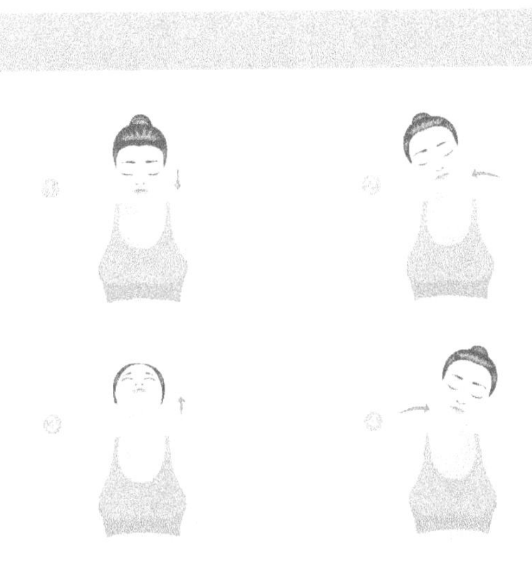

OBJECTIVE OF THE EXERCISE: To relieve tension in the neck and shoulders, improving range of motion and reducing stiffness.

DIFFICULTY LEVEL: Beginner

EQUIPMENT NEEDED: None.

DESCRIPTION:

- Sit in a comfortable chair with your feet flat on the floor.

- Gently lower your chin to your chest, then slowly rotate your head to one side, tilting your head back, then rotating to the other side and returning to your chest.

- The motion should be continuous and circular.

KEY FOCUS POINTS:

- Keep your shoulders relaxed and down away from your ears.

- Move slowly to prevent dizziness.

- Breathe deeply to enhance relaxation while performing the circles.

BENEFITS:

- Reduces neck and shoulder tension.

- Can alleviate headaches related to neck stiffness.

- Helps maintain neck flexibility for daily activities.

VARIATIONS AND ADAPTATIONS:

- For those with limited neck mobility, perform half circles instead, avoiding tilting the head back.

- To increase the stretch, gently place a hand on your head to add a slight pressure.

Frequency and Duration: Complete 3-5 full circles in each direction, once a day.

Objective of the Exercise: To promote flexibility in the hip flexors and quadriceps, which can improve gait and reduce lower back discomfort.

Difficulty Level: Beginner

Equipment Needed: A sturdy chair.

Description:

- Sit on the edge of a chair and hold onto the sides for support.
- Extend one leg out straight in front of you, heel on the floor, then lean forward from the hips, keeping your back straight.

Key Focus Points:

- Avoid rounding the back or slouching.
- Keep the extended leg straight without locking the knee.
- You should feel the stretch along the front of your thigh and hip.

Benefits:

- Enhances hip flexor and quadriceps flexibility.
- Can reduce the likelihood of lower back pain.
- Helps maintain proper posture when walking or standing.

Variations and Adaptations:

- For those with limited flexibility, do not lean forward as much; instead, focus on keeping the back straight and the stretch gentle.
- To deepen the stretch, slightly increase the forward lean while maintaining a straight back.

Frequency and Duration: Hold the stretch for 20-30 seconds for each leg, once a day.

Objective of the Exercise: To relieve tension in the upper back and trapezius muscles, which can result from poor posture or prolonged sitting.

Difficulty Level: Beginner

Equipment Needed: A small towel.

Description:

- Sit in a chair holding a small towel with both hands, then raise your arms above your head.
- Pull on the ends of the towel as you gently bend forward from the waist, allowing your head to move between your arms.

Key Focus Points:

- Keep your neck relaxed and avoid scrunching your shoulders to your ears.

- Bend only as far as comfortable without straining.

- Ensure you are pulling evenly on the towel.

BENEFITS:

- Alleviates tension in the upper back and trapezius.

- Can improve posture and functional movements involving the shoulders and arms.

VARIATIONS AND ADAPTATIONS:

- If raising the arms above the head is too challenging, modify by stretching in front with the towel at chest level.

- To deepen the stretch, widen your grip on the towel as your flexibility increases.

FREQUENCY AND DURATION: Hold the stretch for 20 seconds, repeating 2-3 times per session, once daily.

Calf Stretch with Wall Support

OBJECTIVE OF THE EXERCISE: To stretch the calf muscles and Achilles tendon, improving flexibility for walking and climbing stairs.

DIFFICULTY LEVEL: Beginner

EQUIPMENT NEEDED: A wall.

DESCRIPTION:

- Stand facing a wall with your hands on the wall for balance.

- Step one foot back, keeping it straight, and press the heel down toward the floor.

- Lean into the wall until you feel a stretch in the back leg's calf.

KEY FOCUS POINTS:

- Keep both feet facing forward.

- Ensure the back heel stays on the ground.

- The front knee should be slightly bent.

BENEFITS:

- Improves calf muscle and Achilles tendon flexibility.

- Aids in walking more comfortably and safely.

- Prevents tightness that can lead to discomfort or cramps.

VARIATIONS AND ADAPTATIONS:

- For those who are less flexible, decrease the distance between your feet.

- To increase the stretch, press the back heel firmer into the ground or move the foot further back.

FREQUENCY AND DURATION: Hold for 20-30 seconds for each leg, repeating 2-3 times on each side, once a day.

Embarking on a journey into yoga-inspired balance poses offers seniors an exquisite blend of flexibility and equilibrium. These exercises are meticulously crafted to coax your body into harmony and poise, melding age-old yoga techniques with the realities of a senior's physical capacities. The beauty of these poses lies not in pushing boundaries but in the gentle embrace of one's current abilities, nurturing growth, and confidence. As we explore these serene yet potent postures, remember that each move is a step toward enhanced physical freedom, a beacon of independence, and a testament to the enduring spirit.

TREE POSE VARIATION

OBJECTIVE OF THE EXERCISE: To improve balance and concentration while enhancing leg strength.

DIFFICULTY LEVEL: Beginner

EQUIPMENT NEEDED: None.

DESCRIPTION:

- Stand with your feet hip-distance apart
- Shift your weight onto your right foot
- Place your left foot against the inside of your right ankle, with your knee turned out
- Bring your palms together at your chest or reach your arms overhead for more of a challenge
- Hold for 10-30 seconds, then switch sides.

KEY FOCUS POINTS:

- Focus on a stationary point to maintain balance
- Engage your core to stabilize your posture
- Breathe deeply and evenly throughout the pose.

BENEFITS:

- Builds stability and strength in the ankles and legs
- Encourages mental focus and improves posture.

VARIATIONS AND ADAPTATIONS:

- Place your foot on your shin, avoiding your knee, for a simpler variation
- Use a wall or chair for support if needed.

FREQUENCY AND DURATION: Practice each side 2-3 times, holding for 10-30 seconds per side.

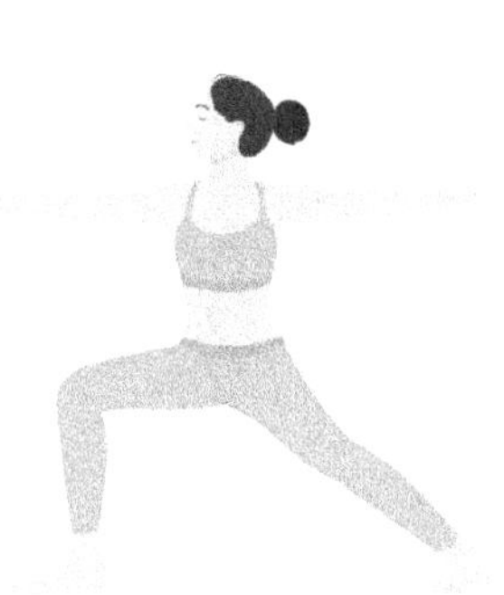

OBJECTIVE OF THE EXERCISE: To strengthen the legs and open the hips, promoting balance and stability.

DIFFICULTY LEVEL: Intermediate

EQUIPMENT NEEDED: None.

DESCRIPTION:

- Start in a standing position
- Step your right foot about three to four feet forward
- Turn your left foot out to a 90-degree angle
- Bend your right knee over your right ankle
- Extend your arms parallel to the floor with palms facing down
- Gaze over your right hand
- Hold for up to 30 seconds and switch sides.

KEY FOCUS POINTS:

- Keep your front knee in line with your foot
- Engage your core and keep your torso straight
- Relax your shoulders away from your ears.

BENEFITS:

- Increases leg strength crucial for mobility
- Enhances concentration and balance.

VARIATIONS AND ADAPTATIONS:

- For an easier version, decrease the bend in the front knee or shorten your stance
- Perform near a wall for additional support if needed.

FREQUENCY AND DURATION: Hold each side for 20-30 seconds, repeating 2-3 times.

OBJECTIVE OF THE EXERCISE: To lengthen the spine and strengthen the arms while providing a sense of grounding.

DIFFICULTY LEVEL: Beginner

EQUIPMENT NEEDED: A chair or stable surface.

DESCRIPTION:

- Place your hands on the seat of the chair or surface
- Walk your feet back until your body forms a right angle
- Let your head hang comfortably between your arms

- Press your hands into the chair and lengthen your spine

- Keep knees slightly bent if necessary.

KEY FOCUS POINTS:

- Keep your weight evenly distributed between your hands and feet

- Actively push away from the chair to deepen the stretch in your spine.

BENEFITS:

- Enhances upper body strength

- Promotes spine flexibility and rejuvenates the body's energy.

VARIATIONS AND ADAPTATIONS:

- To simplify, keep the knees more bent or lift the height of the hands with a higher surface

FREQUENCY AND DURATION: Practice for 30 seconds to 1 minute, repeating 2-3 times.

CHAIR PIGEON POSE

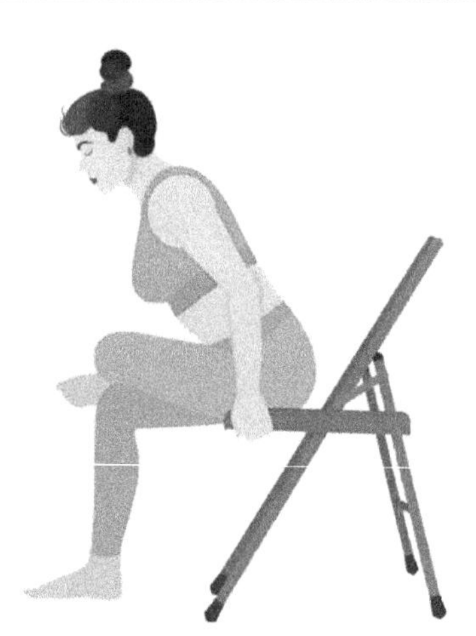

OBJECTIVE OF THE EXERCISE: To open the hips and increase flexibility, reducing tension in the lower body.

DIFFICULTY LEVEL: Beginner

EQUIPMENT NEEDED: A chair.

DESCRIPTION:

- Sit comfortably in the chair

- Cross your right ankle over your left knee, forming a figure-4 shape

- Sit up tall and gently lean forward from your hips to deepen the stretch

- Hold for 20-30 seconds, then switch sides.

KEY FOCUS POINTS:

- Keep your foot flexed to protect your knee

- Maintain a straight back as you lean forward for a proper stretch.

BENEFITS:

- Reduces stiffness in the hips and lower back

- Can aid in preventing sciatic discomfort.

VARIATIONS AND ADAPTATIONS:

- To lessen the intensity, do not lean forward as much

- If flexible enough, progress to a seated floor version.

FREQUENCY AND DURATION: Hold each side for 20-30 seconds, repeating 2-3 times.

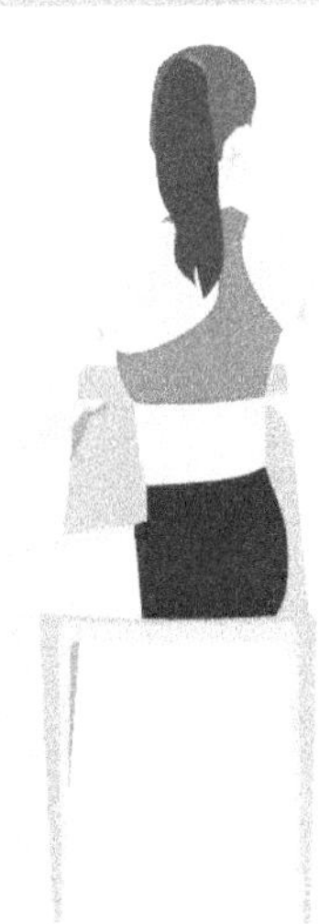

OBJECTIVE OF THE EXERCISE: To enhance spinal mobility and aid digestion, while also nurturing balance.

DIFFICULTY LEVEL: Beginner

EQUIPMENT NEEDED: A chair.

DESCRIPTION:

- Sit on the edge of a chair with your feet flat and knees together
- Turn your torso to the right, placing your left hand on the outside of your right thigh
- Use your right hand on the back of the chair to deepen the twist
- Hold for 15-30 seconds, then switch sides.

KEY FOCUS POINTS:

- Exhale as you deepen the twist
- Keep your spine long and avoid slumping.

BENEFITS:

- Encourages spinal flexibility and can alleviate back tension
- Aids in digestion and internal organ function.

VARIATIONS AND ADAPTATIONS:

- Perform the twist with less rotation for a gentler stretch
- If more mobility is present, twist without the aid of hands for support.

FREQUENCY AND DURATION: Repeat on each side 2-3 times, holding each twist for 15-30 seconds.

OBJECTIVE OF THE EXERCISE: To strengthen the calves and ankles and improve postural alignment.

DIFFICULTY LEVEL: Beginner

EQUIPMENT NEEDED: None.

DESCRIPTION:

- Stand tall with feet hip-width apart
- Engage your thigh muscles and lift your toes, rising onto the balls of your feet
- Bring arms overhead if you can
- Lower your toes back down with control
- Repeat the toe raise motion.

KEY FOCUS POINTS:

- Keep your body line straight, avoid leaning forward or backward

- Engage your core muscles for stability.

BENEFITS:

- Strengthens lower leg muscles critical for walking

- Promotes better body alignment.

VARIATIONS AND ADAPTATIONS:

- Perform the pose seated if standing is too challenging

- For more stability, practice near a wall.

FREQUENCY AND DURATION: Perform 10-15 toe raises, holding each lift for 1-3 seconds.

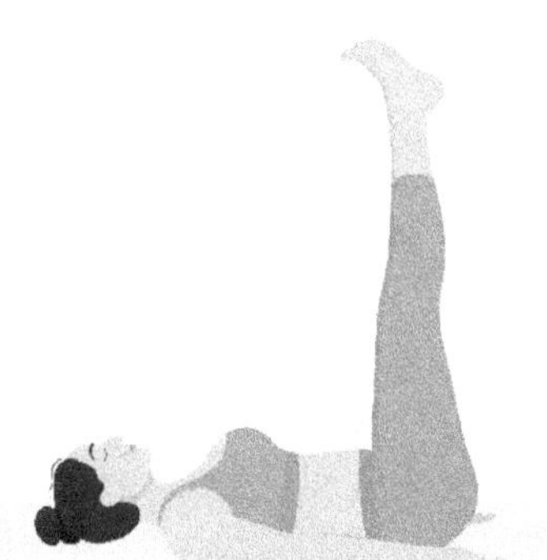

OBJECTIVE OF THE EXERCISE: To relax the mind and body, reduce swelling in the legs, and improve circulation.

DIFFICULTY LEVEL: Beginner

EQUIPMENT NEEDED: A wall space.

DESCRIPTION:

- Sit with one side against the wall

- Swing your legs up onto the wall as you lie back

- Your buttocks can be close to or slightly away from the wall

- Rest your arms out to the sides or on your belly

- Hold for 5-15 minutes.

KEY FOCUS POINTS:

- Support your head if needed to maintain alignment

- Let your legs relax against the wall with a little softness in the knees.

BENEFITS:

- Improves venous return and reduces swelling in the legs

- Calms the nervous system and relieves stress.

VARIATIONS AND ADAPTATIONS:

- For tighter hamstrings, move your buttocks farther away from the wall

- Place a cushion under the hips for elevation.

FREQUENCY AND DURATION: Stay in the pose for 5-15 minutes, depending on comfort level.

Welcome to a series of Pilates exercises meticulously crafted to improve not only your core strength but also your balance. In this carefully selected collection, you, my esteemed reader, will discover the perfect blend of gentle, progressive movements tailored specifically for enhancing the gracious aging process. These exercises are designed not merely for physical conditioning but also for fostering an inner sense of harmony and control. Let's embrace the fluidity and concentration of Pilates to elevate our flexibility and balance to new heights.

Leg Circle

Objective of the Exercise: To enhance hip mobility and core stability.

Difficulty Level: Intermediate

Equipment Needed: Exercise mat.

Description:

- Lie on your back on the mat with one leg extended towards the ceiling and the other flat on the ground.
- Circle the raised leg in a controlled manner, keeping the rest of your body still.
- Switch directions after 5 circles, then switch legs.

Key Focus Points:

- Keep your pelvis stable.
- Engage your core throughout the exercise.
- Keep your movements controlled and smooth.

Benefits:

- Increases hip mobility and stability.
- Strengthens the core and improves coordination.

Variations and Adaptations:

- To modify, make smaller circles.
- For more challenge, increase the size of the circles.

Frequency and Duration: Perform 5 circles in each direction with each leg, twice.

OBJECTIVE OF THE EXERCISE: To enhance core strength, coordination, and balance while stimulating the mind-body connection.

DIFFICULTY LEVEL: Intermediate

EQUIPMENT NEEDED: Yoga mat.

DESCRIPTION:

- Begin by lying on your back with knees bent and arms extended towards the ceiling.
- Inhale and as you exhale, engage your core to lift your upper body and arms toward your knees, keeping your spine curved.
- Pause at the top with control before slowly rolling back down, vertebra by vertebra.
- Focus on a fluid, controlled movement, and maintain a consistent breathing rhythm throughout the exercise.

KEY FOCUS POINTS:

- Concentration on breath and core engagement
- Precision in the curling and uncurling motion
- Fluidity and grace in movement.

BENEFITS:

- Promotes core strength which supports spinal health
- Enhances balance when transitioning from one posture to another
- Encourages mental focus and enhances coordination.

VARIATIONS AND ADAPTATIONS:

- To modify, keep feet on the floor and fold only halfway up.
- For an added challenge, extend one leg at a 45-degree angle from the floor as you curl up.

FREQUENCY AND DURATION: Recommended 5-8 repetitions, once daily.

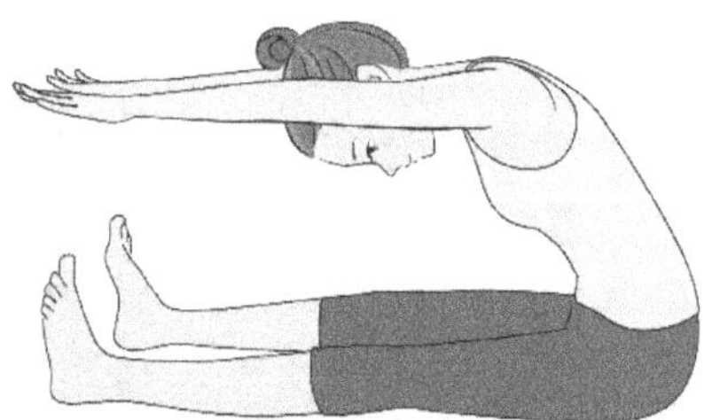

OBJECTIVE OF THE EXERCISE: To increase flexibility in the spine, lengthening the back muscles, and enhancing alignment.

DIFFICULTY LEVEL: Beginner

EQUIPMENT NEEDED: Yoga mat.

DESCRIPTION:

- Sit up tall with your legs extended in front of you, slightly wider than hips-width apart.
- Extend your arms forward at shoulder height.

● Inhale deeply and as you exhale, stretch your spine forward and reach your hands towards your feet, curving your back and dropping your head down.

● Hold the stretch, breathing into the back, then slowly roll back up to a seated position.

KEY FOCUS POINTS:

● Lengthening the entire spine on each stretch

● Keeping the head aligned with the arms as you reach forward

● Engaging the abdominal muscles to support the movement.

BENEFITS:

● Improves spinal flexibility which enhances overall balance

● Relieves tension in the back muscles

● Encourages deep abdominal breathing.

VARIATIONS AND ADAPTATIONS:

● If reaching for the feet is challenging, use a towel or strap around the feet for support.

● For increased intensity, hold the stretch longer, up to 30 seconds.

FREQUENCY AND DURATION: Perform 4-6 repetitions, preferably in the morning to limber up.

PELVIC CURL

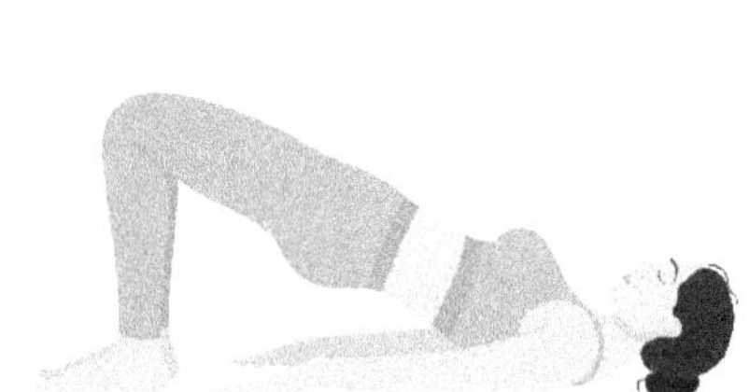

OBJECTIVE OF THE EXERCISE: To increase flexibility in the lower back and strengthen the core stabilizers.

DIFFICULTY LEVEL: Beginner

EQUIPMENT NEEDED: Yoga mat.

DESCRIPTION:

● Begin by lying on your back with knees bent, feet flat on the floor, and arms at your sides.

● Inhale to prepare, and on the exhale, slowly roll your spine off the mat, starting from the tailbone and moving up to your shoulders.

● At the top of the curl, inhale and hold before exhaling to gradually return to the starting position.

KEY FOCUS POINTS:

● Articulating each vertebra during the lift and lowering

● Engaging the buttocks at the top of the curl

● Maintaining the rhythm of your breath to support movement.

BENEFITS:

● Promotes spinal articulation improving flexibility

● Strengthens the glutes and hamstrings which support balance

- Activates the deep core muscles for improved stability.

VARIATIONS AND ADAPTATIONS:

- To decrease intensity, perform the curl only partially.
- For a challenge, at the top, extend one leg toward the ceiling and hold briefly.

FREQUENCY AND DURATION: Aim for 6-8 full curls, twice a day.

OBJECTIVE OF THE EXERCISE: To strengthen the hip abductors and improve lateral balance.

DIFFICULTY LEVEL: Beginner

EQUIPMENT NEEDED: Exercise mat.

DESCRIPTION:

- Lie on your side with your legs stacked and head resting on your lower arm.
- Lift your top leg up while keeping it straight, then lower it back down in a controlled manner.

KEY FOCUS POINTS:

- Keep your hips stacked and avoid rolling backwards.
- Engage your core to maintain stability.
- Move your leg smoothly without jerking.

BENEFITS:

- Strengthens the muscles on the outer thigh and hip.
- Improves balance and stability when walking or standing.

VARIATIONS AND ADAPTATIONS:

- For more comfort, place a cushion under your head.
- To increase difficulty, add ankle weights.

FREQUENCY AND DURATION: Perform 10-12 lifts on each side, once a day.

OBJECTIVE OF THE EXERCISE: To stretch the sides of the body and improve flexibility.

DIFFICULTY LEVEL: Beginner

EQUIPMENT NEEDED: Exercise mat or chair.

DESCRIPTION:

- Sit with your legs folded to one side or sit in a chair.
- Reach one arm overhead and lean to the opposite side, creating a stretch along your side.

- Keep your hips grounded.
- Breathe deeply and elongate your spine as you stretch.
- Move gently into and out of the stretch.

BENEFITS:

- Enhances flexibility in the sides of the torso.
- Helps in reducing tension in the shoulders and neck.

VARIATIONS AND ADAPTATIONS:

- For a deeper stretch, extend both arms overhead.
- To modify, perform the stretch while sitting in a chair.

FREQUENCY AND DURATION: Hold the stretch for 20-30 seconds, repeat 2-3 times on each side.

SAW

OBJECTIVE OF THE EXERCISE: To improve flexibility and rotation in the spine.

DIFFICULTY LEVEL: Intermediate

EQUIPMENT NEEDED: Exercise mat.

DESCRIPTION:

- Sit with your legs wide apart and arms extended to the sides.
- Twist your torso and reach your opposite hand towards your foot, while the other hand reaches behind you.
- Return to the center and repeat on the other side.

KEY FOCUS POINTS:

- Keep your legs grounded.
- Inhale as you twist, exhale as you reach.
- Lead with your chest, not your head.

BENEFITS:

- Increases spinal rotation and flexibility.
- Strengthens the obliques and improves posture.

VARIATIONS AND ADAPTATIONS:

- For a gentler version, bend your knees slightly.
- To increase the stretch, reach further toward your foot.

FREQUENCY AND DURATION: Perform 6-8 repetitions on each side.

CHAPTER 10: EVERYDAY ACTIVITIES AND BALANCE

As we traverse the path of life, the world around us continually shifts and teeters, challenging our stability — a symphony in which we seek harmony between movement and serenity. Dear reader, it's in the dance of our everyday activities, from the moment we rise from our beds to the quiet hours before we retire, that we are presented with a multitude of opportunities to thread the needle of balance into the rich tapestry of daily life.

Embracing Balance with Every Step

Balance is not just a skill reserved for your exercise routine; it's an integral part of every move you make. Imagine turning the mundane, the simple acts of reaching for a book or stepping out to get the mail, into a chance to fortify your foundations of stability. Each daily task holds the promise of becoming a vessel for enhancing your balance.

How often have we passed the kitchen counter, a silent witness to our countless ambles through the heart of our homes? Let it be your comrade in balance, offering support as you march on the spot, feeling the weight shift from the balls to the heels of your feet. With each step, a surge of strength flows through your legs, anchoring you to the earth with the assurance of your own improved agility.

The Symphony of Household Chores

Household chores are a concert of movement; filling the silence with the fluid motion of life within our sanctuaries. As you sweep the floors, be mindful of how you plant your feet before you pivot, turning each sweep into a polished performance of grace. Extend this practice to gardening, where bending to tend the earth also bends the rules of balancing — use one leg as an anchor and the other as a guide, maintaining equilibrium as you nurture life in your backyard Eden.

The act of vacuuming morphs from a mundane task to a dance, the machine a partner in your pas de deux. Push and pull with purpose, maintaining an even distribution of weight, and take pride in the fact that you are not only cleaning but also grounding your sense of physical presence in your environment.

The Art of Culinary Balance

In the culinary ballet of the kitchen, every whisk and chop can grow into an exercise in stability. Engage your core as you reach for spices or stir a pot, allowing the gentle fire of culinary creation to stoke the embers of your inner strength. When standing by the countertop, rise to the balls of your feet and back down, turning a simple wait for the kettle to boil into a chance to elevate your stability practices.

Dining, too, can become an ensemble of balance and poise. Sit at the edge of your chair, feet firmly on the ground, and feel the solid support of your body as you dine. The ritual of the meal thus transforms, nourishing not just the body, but also the spirit of independence that dwells within.

The Realm of Recreation

Leisure activities are the playgrounds for our sense of balance. Engaging in crafts, savor the chance to reach and stretch across your table, extending your range of motion along with your creativity. Should you prefer the company of words, allow yourself the stretch and bend to retrieve a book from a shelf, honoring the wisdom within the pages and your own body's ability to keep you poised.

Game-playing with grandchildren or peers can be a hidden mine of balance work. Stand firm as you throw a ball or extend in a game of catch, finding joy not just in laughter, but in the physical harmony you create with each move. Embrace these moments of connection, for they are the oils that keep the machinery of our limbs supple and strong.

Transforming Errands into Balance Opportunities

Even the act of running errands is an unsung hero in your balance narrative. The walk to the car, the transit from parking lots to doorways, are your stages for a subtle ballet of balance. Walk with intention, aware of how your feet kiss the ground, how your body navigates the shifting terrains. These unwitting rehearsals are acts of defiance against the instability that seeks to upend our confidence.

While shopping, the cart becomes more than a vehicle for provisions; it is a steady partner in your procession down the aisles. Use it to practice standing on one leg briefly as you reach for items, transforming necessity into a serendipitous moment of balance training. With every item that you gently place in your cart, you are lifting not just cans and boxes but the very fabric of your autonomy.

The Quietude of Reflective Balance

Let us not forget the interlude of calmness that punctuates each day — time spent in reflection, contemplation, or pursuing solitary pleasures such as reading. Here, seated in your favorite chair, is an unassuming space for balance exercises. Leg lifts, ankle circles, or even seated marches contribute to the narrative of your day, reinforcing the core and lower body stability that is essential to tackle life's ebbs and flows.

Balance is the Thread We Weave into Life's Tapestry

With each sunbeam that crosses the threshold of dawn to dusk, it becomes evident that balance is not a solitary practice session but an undercurrent in the river of our daily lives. Embracing these opportunities for balance exercises within everyday routines is to exist in a continual state of growth and adaptation. As we gently challenge the boundaries of our physicality with each chore, each moment of leisure, and each small errand, we are writing an audacious story of self-reliance and strength.

In this journey, it is crucial to remember that the pursuit of balance is not about the absence of falls but about the courage to rise and the wisdom to integrate these practices into every step we take. It is the quiet confidence, born from the repeated affirmation that one's own body is a vessel of capable and resilient movement.

As you journey forward, allow the fabric of your day to be stitched with the golden threads of balance, turning every task into a mosaic of movement and poise. Walk this path with the knowledge that each day offers a canvas upon which you paint your independence, one balanced step at a time.

As we journey together through the landscape of balance, we come to recognize that it's not only about exercises done in sets and repeats; it's about weaving balance into the very fabric of our daily lives. Our hobbies and activities—those moments of joy, creativity, and connection—can become rich opportunities to strengthen our balance and, by extension, enrich our quality of life.

In this golden stage of life, the activities we cherish are not just leisurely pastimes; they're gateways to maintaining our independence and mobility. Let's explore how certain hobbies can be delightful allies in our quest for better balance.

Gardening: A Natural Path to Stability

The simple act of tending to a garden is a feast for the senses and the balance system. Reaching for a branch or bending to plant seeds are actions that gently challenge our stabilizing muscles. The uneven terrain of a garden provides a natural environment to practice maintaining our posture. And when we grip a shovel or balance a watering can, we're doing more than cultivating blooms; we're strengthening our resolve to stand firm both in the garden and in life.

Dance: Moving with Grace

Dance is an art form that epitomizes balance in motion. From the gentle sway of a waltz to the jubilant steps of a folk dance, each movement is a testament to the harmony between body and mind. It's an invitation to let the music guide us into a flow of controlled, rhythmic movements that cater to different balance components—timing, spatial orientation, and muscle coordination.

Art and Craft: The Precision of Creation

There's a subtle dance in the brushstrokes of a painter, the delicate threading of a needle by a quilt-maker, or the strategic movements of a sculptor. These creative endeavors engage fine motor skills and concentration, but they also call upon our postural muscles to adapt to various positions as we engage in our craft. By focusing on the detail and precision required for art, we inadvertently give our balance a canvas to improve upon.

Cooking: A Recipe for Equilibrium

Cooking is a sensory-rich experience that also stirs the pot of balance training. Standing at the counter, shifting weight from one leg to the other, or reaching up into cupboards are all actions that recruit balance and stability. The careful coordination required to measure, chop, and stir is not just about creating a delicious meal—it's about nourishing our body's intrinsic ability to stay centered.

Fishing: Patience and Posture Intertwined

Picture the serene environment of a riverbank or seashore—the perfect setting for fishing, a patient pursuit that marries balance and tranquility. Whether we're casting a line from a standing position or maneuvering a boat, we're embracing a practice that encourages us to find our physical footing and anchor our concentration.

Playing Games: Strategy and Stability

Think of games like bocce ball, croquet, or even lawn bowling. They're not simply pastimes; they're strategic games that have us moving in various planes of motion, gauging distances and navigating around obstacles. Beyond the cognitive benefits of strategy, these games offer multifaceted balance practice with every step, every throw, and every intention to win.

Exploring Nature: Step by Step

The great outdoors is a majestic gymnasium for balance. A simple hike or a leisurely walk through a park provides varied terrain for our bodies to adapt to. The subtle adjustments we must make as we step over a root or walk on a trail help keep our balance mechanisms vigilant and responsive. Each time we set out, we're not just sightseeing; we're footing the path to resilience.

Musical Instruments: Harmony in Coordination

Playing a musical instrument, be it as classical as the piano or as folksy as the ukulele, is an impressive display of coordination and balance. The posture we adopt, the control of breath for wind instruments, and the intricate finger movements all work together to create music while concurrently tuning our body's balance system.

Volunteering: A Balance of Giving and Receiving

Engaging in volunteer work is as much a service to our balance as it is to our community. The tasks involved often require gentle physical activity that can improve stability, whether it's wrapping gifts at a local shelter, organizing library books, or walking dogs at an animal rescue. These activities are special—the satisfaction of giving back intertwines beautifully with the physical benefits we receive.

Photography: Capturing Balance in a Lens

Photography—a pursuit of capturing the perfect shot—leads us through various postures and stances. It encourages us to support ourselves effectively as we crouch, lean, or pivot for that ideal angle, all the while honing in on our proprioceptive abilities to hold a steady frame.

Tai Chi: The Art of Moving Meditation

Tai Chi, often described as meditation in motion, is a tranquil yet powerful form of exercise for balance. The slow, purposeful movements accompanied by deep breathing facilitate not just a calm mind but also the subtle strengthening of core muscles vital for balance. Practicing this ancient form of body discipline is a homage to the equilibrium between the internal and the external.

Swimming: The Fluid Dynamics of Stability

While swimming, our body becomes at one with the water, which provides a supportive environment that minimizes the risk of falls. Whether we're performing the breaststroke or simply moving around in the water during an aqua aerobics class, the slight resistance of water furnishes us with an excellent medium for balance and strength training without strain.

In each of these activities, the hidden gem is their capacity to fuse pleasure with purpose. They prove that working on our balance doesn't have to be a mundane routine; it can be interlaced with the richness of everyday experiences, joy, and fulfillment.

As we partake in these hobbies, we're doing more than just filling our time; we're filling our lives with strength, stability, and a newfound sense of freedom. Let's remember, our balance is not only about the ability to stand firm—it's about embracing the rhythm of life while stepping confidently into each new day.

Navigating the great outdoors provides not only a refreshing change of scenery but also a series of unique challenges for maintaining balance and stability. As you step outside, you're greeted with varying textures underfoot—from the soft grass in your backyard to the grainy gravel of a park trail. The uneven surfaces are like life itself—unpredictable and ever-changing. Embracing these natural obstacles can be a joyful exercise in both physical and mental agility.

Let's take a gentle stroll together through the techniques and precautions that can transform your outdoor excursions into safe, enjoyable, and confidence-building experiences.

The Lay of the Land

Visualize an outdoor setting you frequent or wish to visit. Experiencing uneven ground is inevitable—be it sidewalks that have seen better days, garden paths dotted with stones, or park trails with their mélange of soil and roots. Each step on these surfaces is a unique interaction, a dialogue between your body and the earth. Balance, dear friends, is not just about steadiness; it's about adaptability. And outdoors, the art of adapting is paramount.

Adjusting Your Stride

When you encounter irregular terrain, your normal walk might not suffice. Shortening your stride can help. Think of your feet as cautious explorers, each step a gentle inquiry rather than a bold declaration. By taking smaller steps, you lower your center of gravity, giving you a stable base from which to adjust your balance with each new step.

Footwear: The Right Tools for the Walk

This can't be overstated: shoes are critical. You want footwear that hugs your feet snugly, with good arch support and non-slip soles. Shoes that are too loose or lack proper tread can turn an innocent outing into an exercise in hazard avoidance. So, pick your shoes like you would companions for the journey — wisely, and with an eye for loyalty through thick and thin.

Techniques for Tackling Slopes

Slopes can be tricky, but manageable. When you're going uphill, lean forward slightly—it's like telling your body, "I'm with you, let's conquer this hill together." Conversely, when going downhill, lean back just a bit to counteract gravity's pull. Remember, your reliable footsteps are crucial; let the heel hit the ground first, gradually transferring the weight through your foot to the toes.

Using Aids for Extra Support

There's no shame in using a cane or a walking stick—consider these as extensions of yourself, tools to assist in your balance quest. They act as extra limbs, interfacing with the ground to give you additional reference points for stability. When using a cane, plant it firmly before stepping forward with the opposite leg, creating a rhythm that flows with your natural gait.

Staying Present: The Art of Mindful Walking

Amidst the physical aspects of navigating uneven terrain, don't forget the mental component—mindful walking. This involves being fully present with each step, conscious of the sensation of your feet touching the ground, aware of your surroundings and how your body feels as it moves. It's a form of meditation in motion, where you're tuned into the act of walking itself.

Preventing Falls: Anticipation and Reaction

Anticipating changes in the terrain is a skill cultivated through practice. Watch the ground ahead but don't forget to also lift your gaze regularly, taking in the broader path. Should you stumble, react by bending your knees and going with the momentum—a controlled roll can minimize injury compared to a stiff, hard fall.

Taking Breaks: Respect Your Limits

Knowing—and respecting—your limits is a sign of wisdom, not weakness. If you feel fatigued, take a break. Find a bench, a log, or even a large rock to rest on. Use these pauses to reflect on how far you've come, not just on that day's walk but on your journey of balance overall.

Encountering Obstacles: Hop, Step, and Sidle

Different obstacles require different approaches. A high step, such as a curb, might necessitate a gentle hop. Standing firm on the supporting leg while lifting the other knee can achieve this. For narrow passages, side-stepping might be your method of choice, shifting your weight from one foot to the other with care.

Weather and Seasons: Adapting to Change

The seasons turn, and with them, the walking conditions. Ice, snow, wet leaves—each presents its specific challenges. Ice calls for shoes with strong grip or even attachable cleats. Snow suggests a slower pace, whilst wet leaves warn of hidden pitfalls underneath. Respect these seasonal changes; they are part of the ever-dynamic tapestry of the natural world.

Preparedness: The Scout's Motto

Before heading out, plan accordingly. Check the weather, inform someone about where you're going, and carry your phone. Pack a small bag with water, a snack, and perhaps a whistle. It's not about being fearful, but about being prepared.

In conclusion, navigating outdoor and uneven surfaces is a potent way to challenge and improve your balance. Take pleasure in these moments outside, where the symphony of nature plays on and the path beckons with both obstacles and beauty. Approach this part of your journey not with apprehension but with a sense of adventure. It's in the embrace of the uneven, the unpredictable, that we often find our truest sense of balance. Remember, every step outside is a chance to discover more about your capabilities, to connect with the environment, and to find joy in the freedom of movement.

Dear reader, I hope these words light a spark within you to venture forth confidently, to greet the undulating paths of the world not as adversaries but as companions on the road to living a full and balanced life.

Chapter 11: Sustaining Your Balance Long-Term

When we embark on any journey, the initial steps are often filled with enthusiasm and determination. However, as the path unfolds, our footsteps may falter, not because of a lack of resolve, but rather due to the absence of a sustainable rhythm. The journey of maintaining balance is no different, especially as the years of wisdom accumulate. In this segment of our journey together, we'll explore the critical aspect of creating and adhering to a consistent balance routine—an element as essential to your well-being as the steadfast ticking of a grandfather clock.

Consistency: The Heartbeat of Progress

Consistency is the quiet hero of progress. It's the dependable force that, over time, transforms modest efforts into lasting achievements. The commitment to a regular balance routine is vital in sustaining your balance and overall health. Think of consistency not as a monumental daily achievement, but rather as small, steady waves lapping against the shore, each one leaving an imperceptible but undeniable mark upon the sand.

Why Consistency Matters

Consistency reinforces movement patterns in your mind and body, solidifying the connection between them. Like well-oiled gears in a clock, the regular practice of balance exercises ensures that your stability mechanisms function smoothly and efficiently. By regularly engaging in your balance routine, you craft a resilient framework that can better withstand life's unexpected wobbles.

Finding Your Rhythm

Establishing a routine may feel daunting at first, like learning a new dance. However, over time, the steps become second nature. Set aside a specific time each day for your balance exercises, whether it be a quiet morning hour or a reflective evening moment. This scheduling acts not just as a reminder, but as a personal appointment for better health, one that you keep with the same dedication as you would any other important commitment.

Designing Your Balance Ritual

Your balance routine should be as unique as you are. Craft it to complement your lifestyle, preferences, and physical capabilities. As you design your ritual, consider the exercises that bring you joy and confidence. Perhaps balance exercises intertwined with soothing music speak to your soul, or maybe a series of movements performed alongside a window with a view of your garden brings tranquility. Whichever exercises you choose, ensure they're ones you'll look forward to each day.

Creating a Supportive Environment

The environment where you practice your balance exercises should be inviting, free from clutter, and safe. Consider the room where you feel most at ease – this may be the perfect location for your daily practice. The space should also be equipped with any aids or equipment you require to perform your exercises safely, like a sturdy chair for seated exercises or a wall to lean on for standing routines.

Overcoming the Plateau

In every endeavor, there comes a moment when progress seems to slow to a halt—the plateau. It's an inevitable phase, but not an insurmountable one. When you encounter this in your balance routine, recall the progress already made and allow it the space to breathe. This plateau is not a signal to despair, but rather an indication to perhaps adjust the rhythm—add variety or increase the challenge of your exercises gently.

The Power of Adaptability

Flexibility within your routine is as necessary as the routine itself. Life has a way of presenting obstacles—illness, travel, or simply an unexpectedly busy day. When your usual routine is disrupted, adapt. Shorten your exercises, modify them, or even mentally rehearse them. What's important is that your commitment to your balance practice continues unwaveringly.

Social Synergy

The energy drawn from social connections can significantly amplify the effectiveness of your routine. Consider partnering with a friend or joining a community group that shares your dedication to balance and health. Together, you can support each other's journeys, celebrate achievements, and even laugh through the missteps.

Celebrating the Milestones

Your balance routine is a deeply personal narrative woven with countless tiny victories—each one deserving celebration. As your steadiness improves, revel in the newfound ease with which you navigate your environment. Allow the pride you feel in these moments to propel you forward.

The Role of Mindfulness

Embed mindfulness within your routine. As you perform each exercise, attend to the sensations in your body—the gentle tug of a muscle, the solidity of the ground beneath your feet. This mindfulness adds a layer of richness to your practice, deepening the connection between mind and body, and enhancing the sensation of being truly anchored in the present moment.

Inviting Technology To Assist

Do not shy away from technology that may offer support and structure to your routine. There are applications and devices designed to remind you of your daily exercise commitment, track your progress, or even guide you through your exercises. Embracing these technological aids can provide a sense of confidence and companionship along your journey.

Sustaining the Journey

The key to a long-term commitment is to understand that your balance routine is not a finite course with an end point, but an evolving part of your life. As the landscapes of your body and your environment change, so too will your balance practices. Welcome these changes not as roadblocks, but as opportunities to grow and learn—even as a senior, your potential is not static, but dynamic.

In Closing

As you embark on this path to sustained balance, remember that the consistency of your actions builds the foundation upon which all else rests. A consistent balance routine is the lifeline to maintaining your physical freedom, an anchor steadying you amid life's ebb and flow. Celebrate every step, adapt with grace, and above all, remain steadfast in your commitment to this dance of balance—it is, after all, a dance of life itself, ever moving, ever hopeful, and uniquely yours.

11.2 ADAPTING EXERCISES FOR ONGOING IMPROVEMENT

As we embark on the journey of maintaining balance and fostering ongoing improvement in our golden years, we recognize that adaptation is not just a part of life—it's the cornerstone of sustained wellness. Adapting exercises to meet our ever-evolving needs is critical for preserving our mobility and stability as we age.

Adaptation: The Bedrock of Ongoing Improvement

In the sphere of balance exercises, adaptation means tweaking and refining movements to match our current abilities while gently challenging ourselves to reach new heights. It is this delicate dance between comfort and challenge that propels us toward lasting improvement.

Imagine your exercise routine as a garden. Just as you would tend to the plants, providing the right amount of water and nutrients, adjusting to the seasons; your balance exercises require the same attentive cultivation. The care you put in determines the growth you'll see.

Embracing a Dynamic Approach

Our bodies are not static entities—they are dynamic, adapting to stimuli and recovering from setbacks. So our approach to balance exercises must be dynamic as well. This dynamic approach includes listening keenly to what our body tells us—it knows when to push forward and when to take a step back.

Modifying Exercises for Enhanced Safety and Effectiveness

As time passes, what was once an effortless task may become a tad more challenging. And that's okay. The key is to modify exercises to maintain both their safety and effectiveness. For instance, if a certain stance becomes difficult, narrowing or widening your base may provide additional support without compromising the benefits of the exercise.

Progressing with Patience and Persistence

Patience is truly a virtue when it comes to progression in balance exercises. Small incremental changes are more sustainable than large leaps. By gradually increasing the duration or intensity of your routines, you're building the stepping stones for ongoing improvement.

Embracing Technology and Innovations

Technology, when used wisely, can be a great ally. Fitness trackers, for example, can provide insights into your progress and help adapt your exercise routine based on the data collected. Do embrace these innovations as aids in fine-tuning your balance exercises for continual improvement.

Listening to Your Body: A Compass for Adaptation

Above all, your body is your most truthful compass. It tells you when an exercise is too much or when it's time to step up your game. If an exercise causes discomfort beyond the normal 'good burn' of a workout, it likely needs to be adapted. This might mean changing the range of motion, incorporating support like a chair, or adjusting the repetition count.

The Role of Professional Guidance

Though attuned to our bodies, sometimes our perceptions can be subjective. A professional perspective can illuminate aspects we might overlook. Regular check-ins with a physical therapist or fitness instructor can be invaluable for adapting your routine to your current ability level, ensuring exercises are done with correct form, and setting realistic benchmarks for improvement.

Staying Fluid in a Changing Landscape

Let's face it: our bodies will continue to change, often in ways we cannot predict. But the spirit of adaptation is about staying fluid. It means making adjustments—sometimes minor, other times more significant—to accommodate these changes. Reducing the range of motion in leg lifts, using balance aids, or even transitioning to seated exercises are all ways to stay responsive to your body's needs.

Customizing Your Routine: Adaptation at Its Core

Consider each exercise as malleable, able to be sculpted to fit your unique form and function. Customization may mean altering the speed at which you perform an exercise or substituting one movement for another that targets the same muscle groups but feels better on your joints.

Mental Agility: Adapting Your Mindset for Growth

Our mindset plays a crucial role in adaptation. Cultivate mental agility by embracing a mindset of growth. Viewing each adjustment not as a step backward but as an opportunity for growth can transform the way you approach exercise.

The Importance of Ongoing Learning

Stay curious and keep learning. Keeping abreast of the latest research in senior fitness could reveal new exercises or methodologies that could be game-changing for your routine. Be open to experimenting with these new techniques as they may offer the precise adaptations that can propel you forward.

Celebrating Adaptations as Milestones

Every time you successfully adapt an exercise to better suit your needs, it's a milestone—a testament to your commitment to self-care. Celebrating these moments fosters a sense of accomplishment and fuels your motivation to continue adapting and improving.

A Sustained Balance: The Enduring Dance of Adaptation

In conclusion, adapting exercises for ongoing improvement is much like an enduring dance with the rhythm of life. It demands awareness, flexibility, and a willingness to change steps as needed. Your journey of balance is unique, and so too will be the adaptations you make along the way.

As the author of your fitness narrative, remember that each chapter is yours to write. With each adaptation, you are not just reacting to change—you are proactively crafting a narrative of sustained balance and poise. So, embrace the art of adaptation, and may it bring you a newfound sense of freedom, independence, and joy in your golden years. After all, the true balance we seek is not just physical; it's the equilibrium between body, mind, and spirit that keeps us dancing through life with grace and strength.

As we walk the path of maintaining and elevating our balance, it's essential to pause, look back at the terrain we've traversed, and celebrate the milestones we've reached. Such moments of reflection and celebration are not just feel-good markers; they're the lifeblood of sustained motivation and commitment to our health and well-being.

Celebrating Progress: The Why and the How

Celebrating your progress is an integral component of any ongoing wellness plan, especially when improving balance. The journey to better stability and mobility is not always a linear one; it can be peppered with plateaus and occasionally a step backward. Yet, every struggle overcome is a testament to your resilience. Growth is in every effort, not just the triumphs.

Take a moment to consider every instance you caught yourself from stumbling, every exercise that felt a little easier, or even the subtle enhancements in your daily activities. *These are your victories.* However, celebrating isn't only about recognizing success; it's also about acknowledging your dedication and effort. Here's how you can celebrate your progress:

Keep a Balance Diary: Jot down exercises, feelings, and daily activities. Looking back on this diary will showcase your journey, allow for reflection, and serve as a tangible measure of your progress.

Share Your Success: Talk about your achievements with friends or group members. Sharing not only bolsters your spirit but also encourages others on their balance journey.

Reward Yourself: Set milestones and attach small rewards to them – perhaps a new book or a special outing upon mastering a new routine or achieving a personal goal.

Enjoy Complementary Activities: Your hard work has opened doors to activities you might have avoided earlier. Go for that walk in the park or join a dance class. Celebrate your newfound confidence in movement by engaging in joyous activity.

Continually celebrating the small successes along the way fuels a positive feedback loop that perpetuates further achievement—a virtuous cycle of inspiration and progress.

Setting New Goals: A Horizon of Possibilities

Maintaining balance and preventing decline must not plateau into complacency. The act of setting new goals is a declaration of your commitment to a more vibrant and fulfilling life. These goals should be both achievable and stretching, bringing you out of your comfort zone while being realistically attainable. Setting goals is an art in itself, blending aspiration with practicality.

Start with Vision: Envisage where your newfound balance can take you in the future. It could be travel, exploring new hobbies, or improving your performance in activities you already enjoy.

Make It Measurable: Vague goals are hard to realize. Make your goals specific. Rather than "I want to improve my balance", how about "I want to stand on one leg for 30 seconds" or "I want to walk half a mile without assistance"?

Break It Down: Large goals can be daunting. Break them down into smaller, manageable tasks to provide a clear roadmap and a sense of ongoing achievement.

Stay Flexible: As your abilities and circumstances change, so too should your goals. Periodically assess and adjust them to stay aligned with what's possible and desirable for you.

Seek Feedback: Talk to a healthcare professional, a personal trainer, or a balance class instructor to get an external perspective on your goals and progress.

Your goals are deeply personal to you and your unique life; they are not in competition with anyone else's. They're about elevating your quality of life, one step at a time.

Overcoming Plateaus and Renewing Motivation

Even with celebration and new goals, there may come a time when progress seems to stall—a plateau. Don't be discouraged; plateaus are a natural part of any journey of improvement. They are not an end, but a reset point, an opportunity to refine focus.

Renewing your motivation can sometimes be as simple as revisiting the reasons that started you on this path or finding new reasons to continue. Maybe now it's about playing with grandchildren with confidence, or being able to take that dream trip without fear of instability. Recall your successes, no matter how small, to reignite the flame of motivation. And if necessary, seek out new sources of inspiration - perhaps a new class, an exercise partner, or a relevant motivational book.

Creating a Supportive Environment for Continuous Growth

The people in your life and the environment you create around yourself can serve as powerful reinforcement for your balance journey. Engaging with peers who share similar goals can provide social encouragement and accountability. Consider joining a senior exercise group, becoming part of a wellness community program, or even starting a balance club among friends. These groups can be a source of support, enthusiasm, and shared knowledge. They also buffer against isolation and reinforce the joy of collective triumph.

But what if you're advancing well and still experiencing an occasional bout of loneliness or disconnectedness? This is the time to embrace technology as an ally. Online communities, virtual classes, and even video chats with loved ones can bridge the gap. Yet, be patient with yourself, as it may take time to grow comfortable with new technologies. It's another aspect of your balance training—maintaining equilibrium in the digital age.

In Conclusion: Your Pathway to a Balanced Future

Looking forward can be exhilarating when you acknowledge how far you've come and the open road that lies ahead. Celebrating progress isn't just about giving yourself a pat on the back; it's about recognizing and reaffirming the value of the journey you're on. The goals you set pivot on what matters most to you, sprouting from desires and dreams for your life.

As you sustain your balance long-term, build on the legacy of your past successes, and approach your goals with the eagerness of a heart willing to explore and experience life fully. Look at each day not just as another 24 hours but as a canvas of possibilities. Every small step you take is a brush stroke on that canvas, painting a future where better balance literally means a more grounded, joyous, and expansive existence.

Your journey to balance and stability is more than a quest for physical health; it's a pursuit of life—a life lived with zest, with poise, and a steady, confident stride. Let each new goal be a stepping stone to that life, and every celebration a reflection of your unwavering commitment to reach it.

www.ingramcontent.com/pod-product-compliance
Lightning Source LLC
Chambersburg PA
CBHW080847260726
48660CB00009B/3242